THE TEACHING RESEARCH CURRICULUM FOR MODERATELY AND SEVERELY HANDICAPPED

GROSS AND FINE MOTOR

THE TEACHING RESEARCH CURRICULUM FOR MODERATELY AND SEVERELY HANDICAPPED

GROSS AND FINE MOTOR

Prepared by

STAFF OF THE TEACHING RESEARCH INFANT AND CHILD CENTER

H. D. Bud Fredericks
Susan Hanks
Linda Makohon
Chris Fruin
William Moore
Torry Piazza-Templeman
Lynn Blair
Bruce Dalke
Pam Hawkins
Michelle Coen
Suzanne Renfroe-Burton
Carol Bunse
Tina Farnes

Cathy Moses
Jane Toews
Anne Marie McGuckin
Bud Moore
Cheryl Riggs
Vic Baldwin
Roy Anderson
Valerie Ashbacher
Vicki Carter
Mary Ann Gage
Gail Rogers
Bernie Samples

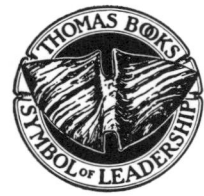

CHARLES C THOMAS · PUBLISHER
Springfield · Illinois · U.S.A.

Published and Distributed Throughout the World by
CHARLES C THOMAS • PUBLISHER
Bannerstone House
301-327 East Lawrence Avenue, Springfield, Illinois, U.S.A.

This book is protected by copyright. No part of it may be produced in any manner without written permission from the publisher.

©*1980*, *by* CHARLES C THOMAS • PUBLISHER
ISBN 0-398-04035-4
Library of Congress Catalog Card Number: 79-26936

With THOMAS BOOKS careful attention is given to all details of manufacturing and design. It is the Publisher's desire to present books that are satisfactory as to their physical qualities and artistic possibilities and appropriate for their particular use. THOMAS BOOKS will be true to those laws of quality that assure a good name and good will.

Library of Congress Cataloging in Publication Data

Fredericks, H D Bud.
   The teaching research curriculum for moderately and severely handicapped.

   Bibliography: p.
   Includes index.
   1. Physical education for handicapped children — Curricula. 2. Motor ability in children — Testing. I. Teaching Research Infant and Child Center. II. Title.
GV445.F73   371.9   79-26936
ISBN 0-398-04035-4

Printed in the United States of America
C-1

ACKNOWLEDGMENTS

THE AUTHORS wish to thank the clerical staff of the Teaching Research Infant and Child Center for their patience and their professionalism in the preparation of this manuscript.

We also wish to thank the Community Mental Retardation Services Section of the Mental Health Division, specifically Mr. David Isom, Mr. Donald Trumbull, Ms. Meredith Brodsky, and Doctor William Fink for their support and encouragement.

Finally, we wish to express our appreciation to the Bureau for the Education of the Handicapped and, specifically, Doctor Ed Sontag for his advice and consultation regarding our early childhood outreach efforts, which partially gave us the motivation to revise our former curriculum and prepare this revised edition.

CONTENTS

	Page
Chapter 1. THE CURRICULUM: ITS BACKGROUND AND USE	3
The History of the Curriculum	3
How the Current Edition Was Developed	3
How the Curriculum Is Organized	4
The Progression of a Student Through the Curriculum	12
The Need to Maintain Skills Once Learned	16
The Need to Use Support Services	16
Summary	20
Chapter 2. PLACEMENT TESTING	21
General Procedures	21
Preparing for the Placement Test	23
Testing Cumulative Skills Programs	25
Where to Begin Testing	25
Reinforcement Procedures	30
Placement Tests	34
Chapter 3. GROSS MOTOR SKILLS	41
A. Lifts Head from Teacher's Shoulder	48
B. Looks at Light	50
C. Attends to Face	52
D. Head Extension on Ball	53
E. Lifts Head While Prone Over Bolster	55
F. Maintains Head Control when Lifted	58
G. Holds Head in Supported Sitting	60
H. Maintains Head in Midline — Supine	62
I. Turns Head — Various Positions	64
J. Bears Weight on Elbows when Placed	66
K. Rolls Side to Back	68
L. Head Righting on Ball — Prone	70
M. Attains and Maintains Weight Bearing on Elbows — Prone	72
N. Follows Moving Objects with Eyes	74
O. Rolls from Stomach to Side	77
P. Bears Weight on One Elbow and Reaches — Prone	79
Q. Rolls from Stomach to Back	81
R. Sits with Support	82
S. Bears Weight on Extended Arms — Sitting	84

		Page
T.	Lifts Head — Supine	86
U.	Rolls from Back to Side	88
V.	Bears Weight on Extended Arms — Prone	90
W.	Pulls to Sit without Head Lag	92
X.	Lifts Head and Shoulders — Supine	94
Y.	Pushed Up on Extended Arms — Prone	95
Z.	Protective Extension Forward on Ball or Bolster	96
AA.	Protective Extension — Forward	98
BB.	Rolls from Side Lying to Stomach	99
CC.	Rolls from Back to Stomach	101
DD.	Weight Bearing with Ball	103
EE.	Sits without Support	106
FF.	Stands with Support	107
GG.	Pivots on Stomach	109
HH.	Lifts Abdomen in Prone Position	111
II.	Bears Weight on Hands and Knees When Placed	113
JJ.	Bears Weight on One Extended Arm and Reaches — Hands and Knees	115
KK.	Moves Toward an Object	117
LL.	Moves Forward Down Ramp	119
MM.	Crawls Forward on Floor	121
NN.	Leans and Regains Balance, Sitting Position	123
OO.	Protective Extension — Lateral	125
PP.	Gets to Sitting from Prone	127
QQ.	Gets to Hands and Knees	129
RR.	Gets to Sitting from Hands and Knees	130
SS.	Pulls to Kneel Stand	132
TT.	Independent Weight Bearing — Grasp	134
UU.	Standing — No Grasp Ability	137
VV.	Lifts Trunk with Hands and Arms	139
WW.	Creeps on Hands and Knees	141
XX.	Turns Trunk in Sitting Position	143
YY.	Gets to Standing from Hands and Knees	145
ZZ.	Gets to Sitting from Supine	148
AAA.	Creeps on Hands and Knees, Negotiating Environment	149
BBB.	Cruises	151
CCC.	Independent Movement — Grasp	153
DDD.	Walking — No Grasp Ability	155
EEE.	Gets to Sitting from Standing	157
FFF.	Sits in Chair	159
GGG.	Gets Up from a Chair	160
HHH.	Falls Forward	161

		Page
III.	Gets into a Chair	162
JJJ.	Walks Up Incline	163
KKK.	Kneels	165
LLL.	Bears Weight on One Knee — Half-Kneeling Position	167
MMM.	Creeps Up Steps	169
NNN.	Rides on Ride-On Toy	171
OOO.	Walks Backwards	173
PPP.	Walks Down Incline	174
QQQ.	Creeps Down Stairs	176
RRR.	Walks Up Stairs	178
SSS.	Walks Down Stairs	180
TTT.	Picks Up Object from Floor — Standing	182
UUU.	Running	184
VVV.	Seats Self at Table	186
WWW.	Rides Tricycle	187
XXX.	Jumps	189
YYY.	Stands on Tiptoes with Eyes Open	191
ZZZ.	Walks Backward on a Line	193
AAAA.	Stands on One Foot, Eyes Open	194
BBBB.	Walks Forward on a Balance Beam	196
CCCC.	Stands Heel to Toe	198
DDDD.	Stands on Tiptoes, Eyes Closed	199
EEEE.	Stands on One Foot, Eyes Closed	201

Chapter 4. FINE MOTOR SKILLS 203
   A. Maintains Grasp on Object — Supine 205
   B. Brings Hands Together — Supine 207
   C. Reaches for Suspended Swinging Objects — Supine . . 209
   D. Reaches for Object — Prone 211
   E. Reaches For and Picks Up, Using Whole Hand Grasp . . 212
   F. Grasps Object with Both Hands 214
   G. Intentionally Releases Object from Grasp 216
   H. Transfers Object from One Hand to the Other . . . 217
   I. Grasps Two Objects, One in Each Hand 219
   J. Reaches For and Picks Up Object, Using Thumb/Fingertips Grasp . 221
   K. Picks Up and Grasps Object, Using Neat Pincer Grasp
      (Thumb and Index Finger) 223
   L. Puts Objects in Small-Mouthed Container 225
   M. Moves Object from One Container to Another 227
   N. Puts Rings on a Peg 228
   O. Builds a Tower 229
   P. Turns Knob 231

		Page
Q. Turns Pages of a Book, One at a Time	.	232
R. Puts Cylinders in Same-Sized Receptacle	.	233
S. Puts Pegs in Pegboard	.	234
T. Strings Beads	.	236
U. Unscrews and Screws on Jar Lid	.	237
V. Pastes Paper	.	239
W. Uses Tongs to Pick Up Objects	.	241
X. Cuts with Scissors	.	242
Y. Laces Ten-Hole Card	.	245
Glossary	.	249
Index	.	251

THE TEACHING RESEARCH CURRICULUM FOR MODERATELY AND SEVERELY HANDICAPPED

GROSS AND FINE MOTOR

In writing this book the authors have chosen to refer to all children as "he," all teachers, aides, and volunteers as "she," and all supervisors as "he." This is done, not to be sexist, but to avoid awkward word formations such as he/she or (s)he. We hope that the reader will accept this style for the purpose for which it was intended — the reader's comfort.

Chapter 1

THE CURRICULUM: ITS BACKGROUND AND USE

THE HISTORY OF THE CURRICULUM

THIS VOLUME is part of the second edition of the *Teaching Research Curriculum for the Moderately and Severely Handicapped*. The first edition, published in 1974, was developed from sequences that were written as individual prescriptions for students. The initial individual prescriptions were then field tested with others and were found to be effective with many of them. A prescribed format was developed, and all sequences were revised accordingly. Thus, the original curriculum consisted of a package of ready-made task analyses that teachers could use in a variety of instructional areas, thereby saving valuable time in the preparation of individual prescriptions.

The first edition of the *Teaching Research Curriculum for the Moderately and Severely Handicapped* was prepared primarily by Ms. Cheryl Riggs and Ms. Torry Furey (Piazza-Templeman). These two individuals did the majority of the work in writing task analyses or adapting sequences that other teachers had written.

The curriculum was used in the Data Based Classroom of the Teaching Research Infant and Child Center. Teachers from throughout the United States were trained in that model, had exposure to the curriculum, and used it in their classrooms. It became apparent as the curriculum was used by more teachers that additional revisions were necessary. Teachers found better ways to organize sequences; they found confusion in some of the sequences that were developed and published; they needed more sequences to be developed; they believed that some sequences could be deleted. Feedback from hundreds of teachers filtered into the Teaching Research Infant and Child Center, and together with the experience of the teachers in the Center, the need for revision of the curriculum became apparent. This is one volume of that revised edition.

HOW THE CURRENT EDITION WAS DEVELOPED

As indicated, the former edition of the curriculum has been tried by many teachers in addition to the teachers in the Teaching Research Infant and Child Center. Moreover, the training staff of the Teaching Research Infant and Child Center who travel widely around the United States had the opportunity to observe the curriculum being used in classrooms in a variety of environments. As a result of the feedback obtained from the teachers who had been trained and due to the work of the staff of the

Infant and Child Center, many of the sequences were designated for revision. In addition, the frequent need for branching some sequences and for preparing additional sequences indicated areas for revision.

The current edition of the *Teaching Research Curriculum for Moderately and Severely Handicapped* was developed by the staff of the Teaching Research Infant and Child Center and Ms. Sue Hanks from the Crippled Children's Division of Oregon, who has been the consulting physical therapist to the Teaching Research Infant and Child Center for the past seven years. Each of the teachers who prepared sections of the curriculum consulted with other teachers, training staff, and consultants to the Teaching Research Infant and Child Center.

Most of the sequences appearing in this edition have been used frequently by teachers in the classrooms with moderately and severely handicapped students. However, it would be misleading to indicate that every sequence in its current form has been adequately field tested with the moderately and severely handicapped population. That has not occurred. In lieu of extensive field testing, which would require many years to complete, the best opinions of teachers and staff who are experienced with this population have been used.

Because our knowledge about the moderately and severely handicapped is continually expanding and because the educational techniques that we develop are ever changing and improving, this curriculum cannot be considered static. Instead, it must be considered dynamic. Those who use this curriculum are encouraged to communicate with the Teaching Research Infant and Child Center to make suggestions about modifications. We welcome those suggestions, and we shall consider them for incorporation in future editions of the curriculum.

HOW THE CURRICULUM IS ORGANIZED

The entire concept of task analysis is based on the premise that a complex skill can be best learned by a student when that skill is broken down into simple, individually taught steps. The curriculum published herein purports to provide that breakdown for skills appropriate to be taught to handicapped children. These are skills that the nonhandicapped child would normally acquire during the first six or seven years of his life but that the severely handicapped child may learn at a later age. Within each skill area, the skills are sequenced in developmental order.

The curriculum is designed to be used in an educational program that designates individual objectives for each student. (A procedure for student placement within the curriculum is recommended in Chapter 2 of this volume.) A student should be placed in the curriculum according to priorities established by the parent and the teacher. The curriculum is designed so that student progress through the various steps of the curriculum can be tracked using a continuous data system. For a complete description of how the curriculum has been utilized in the Data Based Classrooms at the Teaching Research Infant and Child Center, the reader is referred to Fredericks et al., 1979.

The curriculum is organized into curricular areas that include the following: (1) gross motor movements, (2) fine motor movements, (3) receptive language, (4) expressive language, (5) self-feeding, (6) dressing, (7) personal hygiene, (8) table skills, (9) personal information, (10) reading, (11) writing, and (12) number skills. This volume contains gross motor and fine motor skills. Within each of these curricular areas, there are three possible subcomponents called (1) skills, (2) phases, and (3) steps. A skill is a complex behavior requiring the acquisition of a number of subordinate behaviors in order for the learner to achieve mastery. A phase is a further breakdown of a skill. A step is a minute breakdown of the phase.

An example may illustrate how curricular areas, skills, phases, and steps are organized. The following is a task-analyzed sequence within the *curricular area* of gross motor. The *skill* is "Sits with Support." In this instance, the *phases* gradually allow for the removal of teacher support. The *steps* designate the length of time that the student must perform the task.

GROSS MOTOR

R. Sits with Support

Approximate Age for
Skill Acquisition
4-6 months

TERMINAL OBJECTIVE:	Student sits upright, hands free, perpendicular to floor when given support at hips by teacher.
PREREQUISITE SKILLS:	Lifts head prone, bears weight on elbows.
Phase I	Student sits upright, teacher supporting entire trunk, hips and thighs in perpendicular position.
Phase II	Student sits upright, teacher supporting entire trunk and hips in position.
Phase III	Student sits upright, teacher supporting entire trunk, waist to shoulders.
Phase IV	Student sits upright, teacher supporting trunk around ribs.
Phase V	Student sits upright, teacher supporting waist.

Phase VI   Student sits upright, teacher supporting hips.

The following steps apply to all of the phases:

Steps

1. Five seconds.
2. Ten seconds.
3. Fifteen seconds.
4. Twenty seconds.
5. Twenty-five seconds.
6. Thirty seconds.

Variations of the types of phases and steps will occur depending on the type of skills to be taught. This is to be expected since the type of task analysis required varies just as the nature of the task varies.

There are other features on each sequence page. At the top of each page and to the right is a statement that provides the approximate age for skill acquisition. This is the age at which nonhandicapped children usually acquire the skill and represents the best consensus deduced from the developmental literature. A summary of these developmental ages for the sequences in this volume is shown in Table 1-I, the Developmental Chart.

A terminal objective is specified for each sequence. This is the behavior that the student should be able to perform after the sequence has been taught. Prerequisite skills are also designated. Following the phases and steps on each page is a section entitled Suggested Materials. These materials, in some cases, indicate teacher-made materials and in other cases may specify commercial materials readily available in educational marketplaces.

Teaching notes are found at the end of each sequence. In every case, Note 1 is entitled Teaching Sequence. This note is designed to designate the order in which the sequence is to be taught. Since the teaching sequence may vary across programs, the teacher is advised to read the notes carefully. Subsequent teaching notes are designed to give teachers further information, which will allow them to more effectively teach the sequence. A TEACHER SHOULD READ THE ENTIRE SEQUENCE PRIOR TO INSTRUCTION.

A word needs to be inserted here about reverse chaining. Reverse chaining means that the student learns the last part of the task first. For example, when teaching Phase I of the behavior of pasting paper, the student is assisted through the entire procedure, except for the patting of the pasted paper in place, which he is to complete independently. When learning the second phase of the sequence, the student is helped through the sequence, then independently picks up the pasted paper and pats it in

TABLE 1-I
MOTOR

Developmental Age For Skill Emergence	Gross Motor	Fine Motor
1 month	A. Lifts Head from Teacher's Shoulder B. Looks at Light C. Attends to Face D. Head Extension on Ball – Phases I & II E. Lifts Head while Prone over Bolster F. Maintains Head Control when Lifted – Phases I & II	
2 months	D. Head Extension on Ball – Phase III F. Maintains Head Control when Lifted – Phase III G. Holds Head in Supported Sitting – Phases I & II	A. Maintains Grasp on Object – Supine
2½ months		B. Brings Hands Together – Supine
3 months	D. Head Extension on Ball – Phase IV F. Maintains Head Control when Lifted – Phases IV-VII G. Holds Head in Supported Sitting – Phase III H. Maintains Head in Midline – Supine I. Turns Head – Various Positions J. Bears Weight on Elbows when Placed K. Rolls Side to Back L. Head Righting on Ball – Prone M. Attains and Maintains Weight Bearing on Elbows – Prone N. Follows Moving Objects with Eyes – Phase I	C. Reaches for Suspended Swinging Object – Supine

TABLE 1-I *(continued)*

Developmental Age For Skill Emergence	Gross Motor	Fine Motor
4 months	D. Head Extension on Ball – Phase V F. Maintains Head Control when Lifted – Phase VIII N. Follows Moving Objects with Eyes – Phase II O. Rolls from Stomach to Side P. Bears Weight on One Elbow and Reaches – Prone Q. Rolls from Stomach to Back R. Sits with Support	D. Reaches for Objects – Prone
5 months	F. Maintains Head Control when Lifted – Phase IX S. Bears Weight on Extended Arms – Sitting T. Lifts Head – Supine U. Rolls from Back to Side V. Bears Weight on Extended Arms – Prone	E. Reaches For and Picks Up, Using Whole Hand Grasp F. Grasps Object with Both Hands G. Intentionally Releases Object from Grasp H. Transfers Objects from One Hand to the Other
6 months	W. Pulls to Sit without Head Lag X. Lifts Head and Shoulders – Supine Y. Pushes Up on Extended Arms – Prone Z. Protective Extension Forward on Ball or Bolster AA. Protective Extension – Forward	
7 months	BB. Rolls from Side Lying to Stomach CC. Rolls from Back to Stomach DD. Weight Bearing with Ball EE. Sits without Support FF. Sits with Support GG. Pivots on Stomach	I. Grasps Two Objects, One in Each Hand J. Reaches For and Picks Up Object, Using Thumb/Fingertips Grasp K. Picks Up and Grasps Object, Using Neat Pincer Grasp (Thumb and Index Finger)

TABLE 1-I (continued)

Developmental Age For Skill Emergence	Gross Motor	Fine Motor
8 months	HH. Lifts Abdomen in Prone Position II. Bears Weight on Hands and Knees when Placed JJ. Bears Weight on One Extended Arm and Reaches – Hands and Knees	
9 months	KK. Moves toward an Object LL. Moves Forward Down Ramp MM. Crawls Forward on Floor NN. Leans and Regains Balance, Sitting Poisition OO. Protective Extension Lateral PP. Gets to Sitting from Prone QQ. Gets to Hands and Knees RR. Gets to Sitting from Hands and Knees SS. Pulls to Kneel Stand TT. Independent Weight Bearing – Grasp – Phase I UU. Standing – No Grasp Ability – Phases I-IV VV. Lifts Trunk with Hands and Arms	L. Puts Two Objects in Small-Mouthed Container
10 months	TT. Independent Weight Bearing – Grasp – Phases II-III UU. Standing – No Grasp Ability – Phases V and VI WW. Creeps on Hands and Knees XX. Turns Trunk in Sitting Position YY. Gets to Standing from Hands and Knees AAA. Creeps on Hands and Knees, Negotiating Environment BBB. Cruises	

TABLE 1-I (continued)

Developmental Age For Skill Emergence	Gross Motor	Fine Motor
11 months	TT. Independent Weight Bearing – Grasp – Phases IV-VII UU. Standing – No Grasp Ability – Phase VII ZZ. Gets to Sitting from Supine CCC. Independent Movement – Grasp – Phases I and II DDD. Walking – No Grasp Ability – Phases I-IV	
12 months	TT. Independent Weight Bearing – Grasp – Phases VIII-XI UU. Standing – No Grasp Ability – Phase VIII CCC. Independent Movement – Grasp – Phases III-VIII DDD. Walking – No Grasp Ability – Phase V EEE. Gets to Sitting from Standing FFF. Sits in Chair GGG. Gets Up from a Chair	
13 months	HHH. Falls Forward III. Gets into a Chair	
14 months	JJJ. Walks Up Incline KKK. Kneels LLL. Bears Weight on One Knee – Half-Kneeling Position	
15 months	MMM. Creeps Up Steps NNN. Rides on Ride-On Toy	N. Puts Rings on a Peg O. Builds a Tower – Phases I-III
16 months	OOO. Walks Backward PPP. Walks Down Incline	M. Moves Object from One Container to Another O. Builds a Tower – Phases IV-VI
18 months	QQQ. Creeps Down Stairs RRR. Walks Up Stairs – Phase I	Q. Turns Knob

TABLE 1-I *(continued)*

Developmental Age For Skill Emergence	Gross Motor		Fine Motor	
21 months	SSS.	Walks Down Stairs – Phases I-II		
	TTT.	Picks Up Objects from Floor – Standing		
2 years	RRR.	Walks Up Stairs – Phases II-III	P.	Turns Pages of Book, One at a Time
	SSS.	Walks Down Stairs – Phase III	R.	Puts Cylinders in Same-Sized Receptacle
	UUU.	Running	S.	Puts Pegs in Pegboard
	VVV.	Seats Self at Table	T.	Strings Beads
	WWW.	Rides Tricycle		
2½ years	RRR.	Walks Up Stairs – Phases IV-V	U.	Unscrews and Screws on Jar Lid
			V.	Pastes Paper
			W.	Uses Tongs to Pick Up Objects
			X.	Cuts with Scissors
3 years	N.	Follows Moving Objects with Eyes – Phases III, VII, VIII, IX	Y.	Laces Ten-Hole Card
	RRR.	Walks Up Stairs – Phase VI		
	SSS.	Walks Down Stairs – Phase IV		
	XXX.	Jumps		
3½ years	SSS.	Walks Down Stairs – Phase V		
4 years	N.	Follows Moving Objects with Eyes – Phases IV-VI		
	YYY.	Stands on Tiptoes with Eyes Open		
5 years	N.	Follows Moving Objects with Eyes – Phase X		
	SSS.	Walks Down Stairs – Phase VI		
	ZZZ.	Walks Backward on a Line		
	AAAA.	Stands on One Foot, Eyes Open		
	BBBB.	Walks Forward on a Balance Beam		
	CCCC.	Stands Heel to Toe		
	DDDD.	Stands On Tiptoes, Eyes Closed		
	EEEE.	Stands on One Foot, Eyes Closed		

place. The last learned behavior in the pasting sequence is applying paste to the paper (Phase IV). Phases V and VI teach the student to paste within a defined boundary. Thus, in a reverse chain sequence, the student is assisted through all phases that he does not know. In every instance though, he is required to complete the remainder of the task by himself, and at the conclusion of the sequence, patting the paper in place within the prescribed boundary, he would be reinforced.

There are three major advantages to this method of teaching. Since the student is continually reinforced at the same point in the sequence, namely, at the completion of the task, the teacher does not have the problem of fading out the reinforcer at a premature point in the sequence. For example, if the teacher were to use the forward chain process in teaching the task of pasting paper, she would first teach the part of the skill that is designated as "Phase IV — Places drop of paste on paper." When the student mastered that particular task, he would then learn "Phase III — Smearing paste on paper." As he completed this part of the sequence, the teacher would find it necessary to fade the reinforcement at this point and to teach the student "Phase II — Picking up paper with paste." Normally, a student will hesitate after having been reinforced for completing part of the sequence and will wait for the previously delivered reinforcement. The teacher must give an additional cue very frequently in those circumstances and tell the student to continue the task. The reverse chain procedure prevents this difficulty. The second advantage of the reverse chain procedure is that each successive step inherently maintains all previous behaviors learned.

The third advantage to the reverse chain procedure is that, since the student is physically assisted through those parts of the task he is not expected to perform yet, he is exposed to the way in which those behaviors are to be performed and the order in which they occur. Such exposure thereby facilitates acquisition when training of those behaviors commences. When teaching by a forward chain method, this practice effect is frequently lost.

THE PROGRESSION OF A STUDENT THROUGH THE CURRICULUM

The ability to learn a skill is viewed on a continuum. On one end of the continuum is the ability to engage in independent problem solving. On the other end of the continuum is the ability to learn small parts of a task one at a time by systematic withdrawal of assistance.

The ability of most people to learn falls somewhere along that continuum. If the learning environment is effective and motivating, one's ability to learn will progress along the continuum.

When establishing cueing and assistance procedures, the teacher must determine at which point on the continuum the student functions in order to provide a learning environment appropriate to each student's ability to learn.

The task analyses and teaching strategies outlined by this model provide the basic starting point for shaping skills in a systematic and structured way. Some students may require less assistance and less analysis of the task.

The curriculum is designed for a moderately or severely handicapped student. However, the curriculum has been utilized with students who are not as seriously handicapped and has even been used with nonhandicapped preschool children. In these cases, the detailed breakdown into steps may not be necessary, and in some instances, a breakdown of phases may not be necessary. For example, in the gross motor skill of "Stands on One Foot," a less severely handicapped person or a preschool nonhandicapped student may merely require someone to model the behavior for him or to provide a small amount of balancing assistance through the detailed breakdown of phases and steps.

The teacher who uses this curriculum should always have the student attempt to accomplish the terminal behavior of the skill first. (See Chapter 2 for baselining procedures.) If the student is unable to perform the terminal behavior, the individual phases may be taught. Likewise, the teacher should also always try to have the child accomplish a phase at its terminal step before teaching each step of that phase. *There may not be a need to move every child through the curriculum step by step and phase by phase.* A student's progression through the curriculum should depend upon his abilities and the rate at which he can acquire the skills being taught.

On the other hand, the student who is much more handicapped may need a further breakdown of the curriculum. In such a case it is necessary to use a branching technique. Branching refers to the adding of additional steps or phases to the programs. For example, one curriculum sequence teaches a student to walk forward on a balance beam without stepping off. The program reads as follows:

BBBB. Walks Forward on a Balance Beam

Approximate Age for Skill Acquisition
5-7 years

TERMINAL OBJECTIVE: Student walks forward on a balance beam for a distance of 8 feet without stepping off.

PREREQUISITE SKILLS: Walking.

Phase I Student walks forward on 1-foot square rubber mats placed in a straight line.

Phase II Student walks forward on 1-foot square rubber mats staggered so that upper right-hand corner of one mat touches lower left-hand corner of second mat, and so on for eight mats.

Phase III Student walks forward on 4-inch wide tape line, placing heel of one foot against toe of other foot.

Phase IV Student walks forward on 1-inch wide straight line, placing heel of one foot against toe of other foot.

Phase V Student walks forward on 2- by 4-inch board placed on the floor.

Phase VI Student walks forward on balance beam placed on the floor.

Phase VII Student walks forward on balance beam raised 2 inches from floor.

Phase VIII Student walks forward on balance beam raised 4 inches from floor.

Phase IX Student walks forward on balance beam raised 6 inches from floor.

The following steps apply to each of the phases:

Steps
1. Distance of 1 foot without stepping off.
2. Distance of 2 feet without stepping off.
3. Distance of 3 feet without stepping off.
4. Distance of 4 feet without stepping off.
5. Distance of 5 feet without stepping off.
6. Distance of 6 feet without stepping off.
7. Distance of 7 feet without stepping off.
8. Distance of 8 feet without stepping off.

The following example illustrates branching. The student has been successfully taught Phase IV, Step 8. However, he cannot perform Phase V, Step 1 because he seems to be somewhat frightened by the height of the balance beam. The teacher chooses to branch the program by providing the student support. The branches read as follows:

Phase V   Step 1a. Distance of 1 foot without stepping off, with teacher holding both hands.

Step 1b. Distance of 1 foot without stepping off, with teacher holding one hand.

Step 1c. Distance of 1 foot without stepping off, with teacher lightly holding elbow.

Thus, a branch adds additional task analyses to a sequence. In the example shown previously, an additional physical prompt has been added. Verbal prompts can be added in the same manner. These are very common types of branching techniques. Another type of branching is making the step smaller. For instance, in the skill of "Head Extension on a Ball" in the gross motor curricular area, the steps are shown in seconds as follows:

Steps

1. Two seconds.
2. Four seconds.
3. Six seconds.
4. Eight seconds.
5. Ten seconds.
6. Thirteen seconds.
7. Sixteen seconds.
8. Twenty seconds.
9. Twenty-five seconds.
10. Thirty seconds.

Perhaps a student is able to accomplish Step 1 but cannot do Step 2. An appropriate branch would be the following:

Step 1a. 3 seconds.

Despite the fact that the branching of programs may at times be necessary for certain students and that other students may be able to skip entire phases and steps, it is believed that the basic curriculum provides a good foundation for those programs. If branching is required, only a few steps usually need to be written or added to the existing program to modify it to provide a suitable program for a particular student. Thus, the purposes of the curriculum — to save teacher time and to provide a guide — are still achieved.

As indicated earlier, the curriculum is designed to be used with a continuous, or at least very frequent probe, data system. A description of such a data system is provided in Fredericks et al., 1979.

THE NEED TO MAINTAIN SKILLS ONCE LEARNED

A word of caution must be given to the teacher who uses this curriculum. One of the major concerns for teaching a severely handicapped student is the maintenance of his acquired skills. It is natural to forget a skill through disuse. This happens to all people, and it will also happen to the severely handicapped student; therefore, a continual system of review must be incorporated into any teaching environment.

There are two basic types of skills included in the curriculum — cumulative and discrete. A cumulative skill is one that is built upon skills previously learned and that is also incorporated into skills to be learned. A cumulative skill does not require continuous review to be maintained because it will be embodied in future skills that the student learns. A discrete skill will need a system of review to be maintained. For instance, standing is a skill that is cumulative in that, after the student learns how to stand, he probably will be taught to walk. Once he begins walking, there is no need to review his ability to stand. It is embodied in the walking behavior. Almost all motor behaviors are of this character. Once learned, the natural motor movements of the individual will maintain them.

Some skills, however, are discrete in the sense that, if they are not used, there will be some loss of dexterity, coordination, and balance. Walking on a balance beam and cutting with scissors are two examples. However, it is a truism that once a motor behavior is learned it will be retained. A person never forgets how to ride a two-wheel bike, to roller skate, or to throw a ball. Lack of practice may affect the individual's ability to "go fast" or throw accurately, and one may be a little more cautious on roller skates, but a few minutes of practice quickly resurrects the unused skill.

However, it is important that the teacher is confident that the natural environment provides the opportunities for the student to use his newly acquired motor skills. If a student has learned to walk, he should be required to walk and not be carried or allowed to crawl. There must be close coordination between the school and the home to ensure that the learned motor behaviors are being used and to ensure that only the degree of assistance necessary is being provided. The burden of communication to effect this coordination is on the teacher, for she is conducting the instructional program and is most aware of the student's current progress and status in the program.

THE NEED TO USE SUPPORT SERVICES

It must be remembered that the programs written herein are intended as a framework or a guideline for the programming of a given student and can be modified to fit the student or the situation. If necessary, assistance in modification of these programs can be supplied by various support services. In fact, *the utilization of the support services for the severely or profoundly handicapped student should be a mandatory part of his program.* The myriad of skills and techniques for dealing with the diverse problems these students present continues to evolve. No one discipline can realistically embody them all. Educators, speech therapists, physicians, physical therapists, occupational therapists, psychologists, nurses, visual trainers, and all other areas of expertise may be vital to the development of the student's abilities.

The traditional role of professionals in support services has been direct intervention (removal from class for therapy). Although this may be appropriate (and possibly practical) for an occasional student, maximum effect of intervention for a student cannot be achieved unless the objectives and techniques of the expert can be extended to daily use in the classroom and/or home. *When making contact with support services, the educator must make it clear that what is wanted is information to be utilized in developing classroom and/or home programs.* "For example, rather than providing a student with a brief period of therapy each week, the physical therapist trains the teacher and/or parent how to lift, carry, position, and exercise the student" (Bricker, 1976). The teacher of the severely handicapped must become an educational synthesizer. She must learn how to "draw relevant information from a variety of sources and then incorporate it into daily intervention procedures for children" (Bricker, 1976).

There are also other considerations that the classroom teacher must take into account. Failure to utilize expertise when it is available or attempting to fill a role for which one is neither trained nor licensed may well leave the professional open to charges of negligence or malpractice and subsequent law suit. While it is largely the medical field that has been plagued with law suits, the teacher of the multiply handicapped, as they deal more with what have traditionally been considered medical problems, may well be faced with similar difficulties. Utilizing other professionals as consultants is one way to reduce the likelihood of this problem occurring.

Certain ethics and laws apply to utilization of professionals. Although the ethics are not as binding as laws, failure to respect them may produce a highly embarrassing, if not harmful, situation.

Legally, referral of a student to medical, paramedical, or other direct care personnel cannot be made without the knowledge and consent of the student's parent or legal guardian. If a problem has been uncovered that requires the attention of a physician, the parent should be the one to make the contact.

The following are some ethical considerations for the use of support services: Physicians practicing in a specialty should be contacted by the student's pediatrician, family doctor, or parent. A nurse may see a student for evaluation of a problem, but a doctor's referral for specific treatment is required. A physical therapist requires a physician's referral to see a student for evaluation and/or treatment. Direct referral may be made to speech pathology, visual training, psychology, social work, audiology, and occupational therapy. Any of these individuals may request additional information from the student's physician prior to the delivery of service. If a professional is seeing a student, it is considered unethical to request another individual of the same profession to see the student and/or intervene without all parties being aware of the previous involvement.

Table 1-II is a partial list of what should be "red flags" to the educator and of which medical or allied medical services might provide assistance. The left-hand column indicates signs, symptoms, and behaviors that if evident in a student, may interfere with or prevent his education. While they may be undesirable behaviors, they may not be amenable to behavior modification techniques for their remediation. Examples of such behaviors are physiological conditions present in the child, such as spasticity (stiffness), tongue thrust, seizures, sensory deficiencies, etc.

The Teaching Research (TR) classroom model is one which a public school can adopt. The budget under which the TR classrooms operate is similar or less than budgets for similar classrooms located in a public school setting in Oregon. Therefore, TR cannot afford to have on staff the specialists to which students must occasionally be referred. Most school districts also cannot afford that kind of staff on a permanent basis. Consequently, specialists who are used frequently at TR are retained on a consultant basis. For instance, the physical therapist is retained on a consultant basis and visits the center one or two times a month. This interaction is sufficient because of the way in which this consultant is used. She evaluates and recommends programs for those students for whom physical therapy has been indicated by a physician. Recommendations for physical therapy are in programmatic form, and the teacher and the parent of the student for which a recommendation has been written are taught by the therapist how to conduct the program. A data system to measure the progress of the student through the program is established and incorporated into the existing data methodology at TR. These data and the progress through a program are then shared between the home, school, and physical therapist, and the program is updated in the same manner as other programs for the student. If difficulties in a particular program are manifested before the next visit to the therapist, the therapist can be reached by telephone for consultation.

This method of consultation has been used at TR for the past four years. It has quite adequately served all the students in the Center. An analysis of why it has been successful must conclude that the consulting specialists have been able to communicate their programs in a sequenced format, have been responsive to data, and have supported the concept that parents

TABLE 1-II

"RED FLAGS" THAT INDICATE THE NEED FOR SUPPORT SERVICES

IF THE STUDENT –	SEEK ASSISTANCE FROM –
Is excessively stiff or excessively floppy, Is diagnosed cerebral palsy,	Pediatrician, Orthopedist, Physical Therapist, Occupational Therapist (through Physician).
Jerks, stares, twitches, or "blanks out,"	Neurologist.
Chokes easily, pushes food out with his tongue, bites spoon, grimaces repeatedly, opens mouth very wide, remains on baby food after one year chronological age,	Speech Pathologist. Occupational Therapist. Physical Therapist (through Physician).
"Can't get words out," mispronounces sounds, breathes strangely while speaking,	Speech Pathologist.
Shows decided hand preference before age three, Has fisted hands, Becomes very stiff when attempting to use hands, Can't get hand to mouth,	Occupational Therapist and/or Physical Therapist (through Physician).
Has braces, crutches, walker, wheelchair,	Orthopedist, Physical Therapist (through Physician).
Has behavior problems so severe that the classroom teacher can't remediate, Is exceedingly fearful, Shows extreme scatter of abilities,	Psychologist. Nurse.
Is known to be visually impaired, Fails to make eye contact, Fails to follow object with eyes, Fails focus on objects, Fails to smile at Mom's face (no sound),	Ophthalmologist. Visual Trainer.
Fails to have well-established head control by three months,	Physical Therapist (through Physician). Neurologist. Ophthalmologist and/or Visual Trainer.
Has chronic discharge from ears or fusses and holds ears, etc., Does not respond to noise or voice, Talks through his nose, Is known to be hearing impaired,	Otolaryngologist (ENT) or Otologist. Audiologist. Deaf Educator.
Has joints that move abnormally, Has foot, back, or other obvious deformities, Can't spread knees apart 18-24 inches, Is very stiff,	Orthopedist.
Has upper respiratory congestion, Is hyperactive or sleepy, Has skin rashes, Has sores that do not heal, Has seizures, Has poor hygiene, Seems too thin (nutrition), Has behavior problems with toilet training,	Nurse.
Self-stimulates,	Ophthalmologist. Psychologist.
Has normal or borderline IQ, but is tactilely defensive – severe, Has obvious dizziness or balance problems, Has trouble in right/left discrimination, Has no established hand preference after five years, Has severe distractability, Has extreme problems with dressing or feeding, Becomes stiff while feeding or dressing,	Occupational Therapy.

and teacher are capable, after instruction by the consultant, to conduct many of the programs prescribed.

SUMMARY

This chapter has provided a brief history of the development of the curriculum. The organization of the curriculum has been discussed. This chapter has emphasized the need for frequent monitoring of the student's progress through the curricular programs and suggested ways that the curriculum can be modified to accommodate the type of progress the student is making. The importance of monitoring the maintenance of learned skills has been discussed. Finally, the need for effective utilization of support services has been emphasized.

REFERENCES

Bricker, D.: Education synthesizer. In Thomas, M. Angele (Ed.): *Hey, Don't Forget About Me.* CEC Information Center, 1976.

Fredericks, H. D., Baldwin, V. L., Moore, W., Piazza-Templeman, V., Grove, D., Moore, M., Gage, M. A., Blair, L., Alrick, G., Wadlow, M., Fruin, C., Bunse, C., Makohon, L., Samples, B., Moses, C., Rogers, G., Toews, J.: *A Data Based Classroom for the Moderately and Severely Handicapped,* 3rd ed. Monmouth, Instructional Development Corporation, 1979.

Chapter 2

PLACEMENT TESTING

GENERAL PROCEDURES

THE PLACEMENT TEST, which pinpoints as accurately and efficiently as possible in each area of the curriculum the student's acquired skills and deficiencies, is used to determine program placement. Skills are tested by requesting the student to complete the task specified in the terminal objective of the program for a maximum of three trials. Separate trial data (X = correct; 0 = incorrect) are recorded on the placement test form. Pass criterion for each test item is two correct responses out of three possible trials. If the student passes, the teacher records a "yes" adjacent to the corresponding program on the placement test form. If the student responds correctly on only one of the trials or not at all, he has not sufficiently demonstrated mastery of the skill and a "no" is recorded.

Providing a model or demonstration of the task is suggested for skills acquired up to the developmental age of two years and for skills that may not be demonstrated by a student because he fails to comprehend the verbal cue. The purpose of the placement test is to measure whether or not a student can perform a particular skill, not his receptive understanding of the cue (except, of course, for a language placement test). Consider, for example, the program "Grasps Object, Using Neat Pincer Grasp." The student would not be able to understand the particular way you wanted him to grasp the object only from the cue "Pick it up." If he were, in fact, capable of the task, the placement test might not reflect this ability if a model was not provided. Therefore, students in a placement test situation will benefit from a model presentation.

To avoid a possible aversive situation for the new student, the testing session should not be unduly long. Several test sessions with frequent free time breaks, possibly over several days, may be necessary depending on the attention span and skill level of the student.

In order to provide comprehensive programming, it is presumed that most students will be placed in each area of the curriculum, namely, fine and gross motor skills. Therefore, both curricular areas should be placement tested. Also, when the student's Individual Education Plan is rewritten at the beginning of each school year, placement testing should be conducted again. To assist in the process of placing the student in the various components of the curriculum, a placement test for each component has been developed and is presented here.

After having placed the student, the teacher occasionally finds that the

TABLE 2-1
TEACHING RESEARCH PLACEMENT TEST

MOTOR SKILLS

	Program and Suggested Cue	Placement Test				Baseline		Posttest		Comments
		Trial	Data	Yes/No	Date	Data	Date	Data	Date	
P	Turns pages of a book, one at a time – "Turn the page." (model)			Yes*	9/15/78					
Q	Turns knob – specific to materials used – Example: "Open the door"; "Turn it on."			Yes*	9/15/78					
R	Puts cylinders in same-sized receptacle – "Put them in."			Yes*	9/15/78					
S	Puts pegs in pegboard – "Put them in." (model)	X	X	Yes	9/15/78					
T	Strings beads – "String the beads." (model)	O	O	No	9/15/78	0/8	9/10/78	8/8	10/24/78	
U	Unscrews and screws on jar lid – "Open." (model)	O	O	No	9/15/78	1/13	11/2/78	5/13	12/13/78	
V	Pastes paper – "Paste it on." (model)	O	O	No	9/15/78					
W	Uses tongs to pick up object – "Pick it up." (model)									
X	Cuts with scissors – "Cut out the circle; stay on the line." (model)									
Y	Laces ten-hole card – "Lace the circle." (model)									
U(1)	Removes cap from toothpaste			No	12/14/78	0/20	12/14/78	20/20	1/27/79	

* Information obtained from parent/former teacher conferences or informal classroom observations.

placement has been erroneous. One should not be afraid to make adjustments in placement as better evidence of the student's capabilities becomes available.

Programs not included in the curriculum that are written by the teacher to provide individualized programming specific to a particular student's needs may be written in on one of the blank lines following each curricular area. See Table 2-I for an example. Note that the program is assigned the letter U(1). This indicates that it was taught after program U.

PREPARING FOR THE PLACEMENT TEST

Before the placement test is conducted, two steps must be taken:

1. *Allow time for adjustment:* Allow adequate time for the student to adjust to his new environment. This is an important factor since a student's skills may be inhibited or altered by the fact that he is in an unfamiliar setting. The amount of time needed for a student to adjust to the new environment varies with the individual. It is up to the teacher to be sensitive to the new student's ability to feel at ease. Some indications of adjustment are the new student's allowing adults/peers to approach him without withdrawing, approaching others to communicate a need or gain affection, actively participating in the structured group activities, or engaging in free play activities with peers. In the Teaching Research classrooms the usual adjustment time is approximately one to two weeks.

2. *Obtain information:* Gather as much information about the student as possible through conferences with parents and former teachers and by observing closely the student's behaviors in the classroom. The conferences can provide information about the behaviors the student may exhibit in a familiar setting and about the items that are effective reinforcers (favorite toys, food, social praise, tokens, etc.). By informally observing the student's behaviors in the classroom, the teacher is able to more accurately determine a point at which to begin placement testing. During the initial adjustment period, the teacher can also identify possible reinforcers by observing what toys, food, events, people, etc., the student enjoys the most. These will be needed to reward the student for good behavior and "working hard" during the placement test.

STIMULATION TESTING

If the teacher is not able to find out from the parent conference or through informal observation what reinforcers are appropriate for the student, then she can conduct stimulation testing to identify possible reinforcers. A brief description of stimulation testing follows:

The student is presented a series of stimuli designed to appeal to one of the five senses. The purpose of the presentation is to evoke a response from the student. The teacher or therapist observes the student's re-

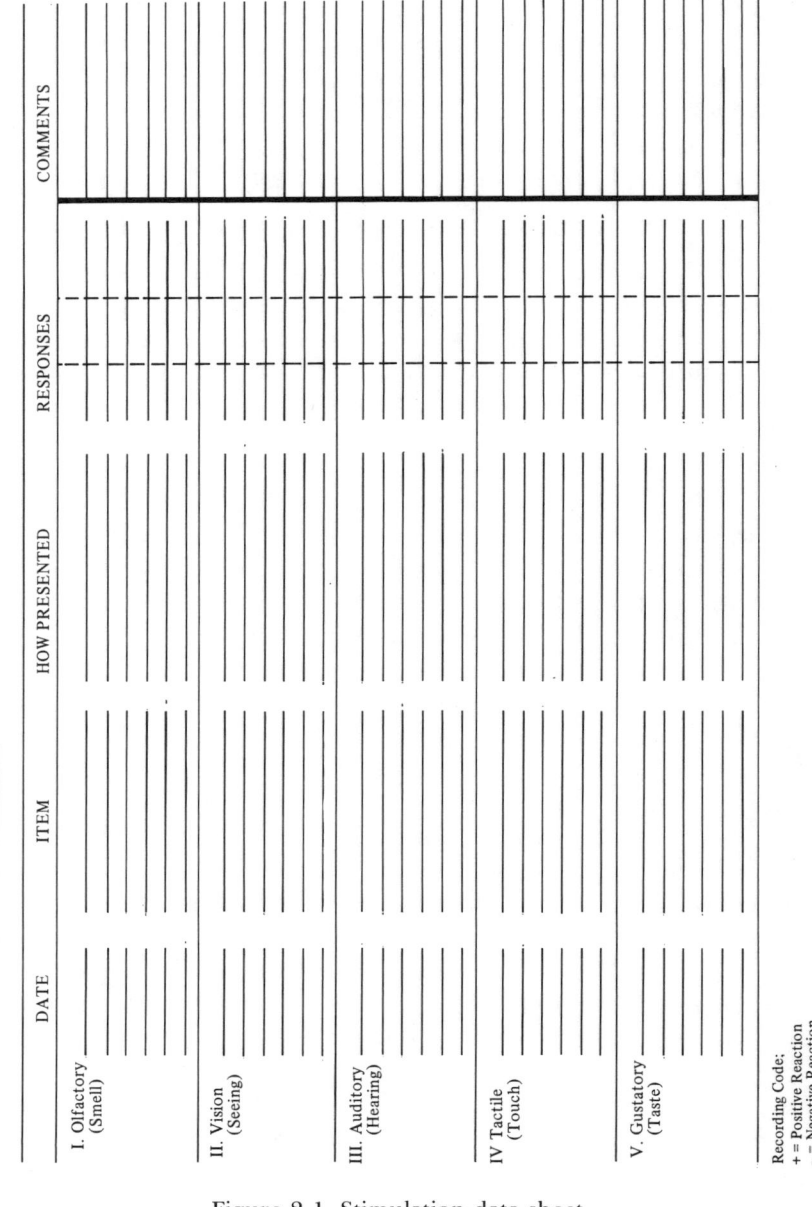

Figure 2-1. Stimulation data sheet.

sponses and records whether the response indicates that the stimulus is pleasing (+) or not pleasing or aversive (−). If the observer is unable to determine in which category the response can be placed but is certain that a response did occur, a (?) is recorded. If no response occurred, a (0) is recorded. See Figure 2-1 for an example of a stimulation form. Consistency of response is needed before a determination is made whether a stimulus is punishing or reinforcing. Three consecutive consistent responses are required over a period of three days. If that consistency is achieved, the stimuli can be said to be a potential reinforcer or punisher. Of course, whether or not a stimulus actually functions as a reinforcer or punisher is determined by its ability to effect a change in behavior.

The teacher should keep in mind that, for profoundly handicapped students and very young children, reinforcers vary considerably. This variation implies that the reinforcers may need to be changed frequently to be effective.

TESTING CUMULATIVE SKILLS PROGRAMS

Cumulative skills programs are those which teach one terminal behavior; the phases and steps of that program build up to that one terminal goal. All the sequences in the motor development curriculum are cumulative sequences. When placement testing a cumulative skill, such as "Strings Beads," it is only necessary to test at the most difficult step of the task analysis. When teaching a skill such as this, it is necessary to acquire Step 1 of the skill before one can go on to Step 2. With each new step of the program, the student is required to perform a greater portion of the task independently. Therefore, if the student can perform Step 4 (most difficult step) independently, it is assumed he can perform the simpler steps (1 through 3). If a student cannot complete Step 4 independently and needs a great deal of assistance, record "no" on the placement test form next to the skill "Strings Beads." It would not be necessary during placement testing to test the other three steps in the program since the placement test is a gross assessment of the student's skills. More specific testing of steps in the program will occur during baselining procedures, which pinpoint the exact phase and step at which to begin teaching a skill.

WHERE TO BEGIN TESTING

Information gathered about the skills of the student from parents, from former teachers, and through informal observations prior to placement testing will provide a point at which to begin testing in each curricular area. In the example provided in Table 2-I, the teacher had informally observed during the adjustment period that the student was able to turn the pages of a book one at a time, open a door (turns knob), and put ten cylinders in the same-sized holes. Thus, the teacher began testing at program S, "Puts Pegs in Pegboard," of the Fine Motor area. Skills that follow on the placement test were then tested until the student did not meet criteria on three skills. Also, any skills preceding the first skill tested about which the teacher has insufficient or no information should be tested.

The bracketing procedure is used for those curricular areas for which the teacher does not have sufficient information to identify a starting point for placement testing. Bracketing provides an efficient determination of program placement because it is a procedure that avoids the need to test every sequence in a particular curricular area.

Begin by dividing the curricular area into sections of about eight to ten skills, grouping the skills by the developmental age norms such that skills occurring between one and two years are in one section, two to three years in another, and so on. The teacher should then be able to determine in which section to begin testing with the student.

Bracketing is a process whereby skills are tested at the end, beginning, and middle points of each section. Final determination of possible programs for placement depends on whether the student passes or fails at those points. Refer to Figure 2-2 for the flow chart for bracketing procedures.

Begin by testing the last skill in the section. If the student passes, test within the next section that follows by testing the last skill in that section first. If the student fails the skill at the end of the section, test the skill at the beginning of the section. If the student fails at that point, test the skills that follow until the student fails three skills. If, however, the student meets criterion on the skill tested at the beginning of the section, test a skill in the middle of the section. If the student fails this middle skill, then his level of performance probably lies somewhere between the beginning and middle; the teacher then tests those skills from the beginning to the middle points of the section until the student fails three skills. If, however, the student passes the middle skill, his abilities probably lie between the middle and end points of the section; thus, the teacher tests the skills that follow the middle skill until the student fails to meet criterion on three skills.

In the example in Table 2-II, testing began with the skill at the end of Section I, "Maintains Head in Midline." Since the student met pass criterion on Skill H, Section II was tested starting with the last skill (0), "Rolls from Stomach to Side." When the student did not demonstrate the ability to perform that task, the teacher tested the first skill in Section II, "Turns Head — Various Positions." When the student passed this skill, the teacher then tested the skill in the middle of Section II, "Head Righting on a Ball." Since the student was not able to perform this task, the teacher then tested Skills J and K. Because the student passed Skill K, the teacher continued by testing Skill M. Failure to pass Skill M provided three "nos" and therefore

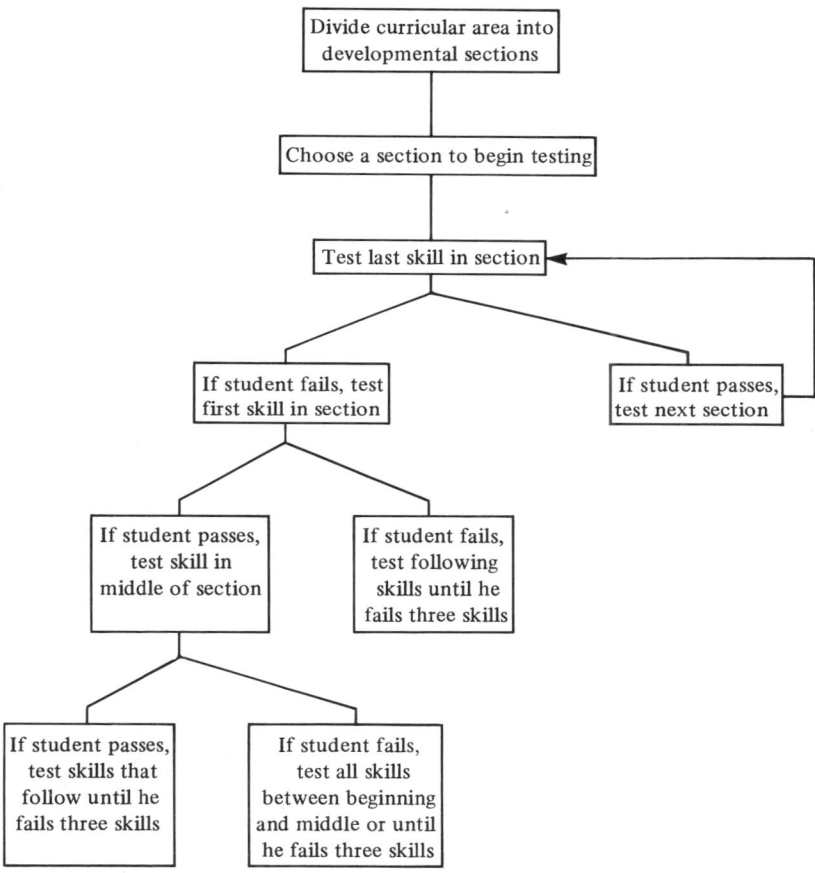
Figure 2-2. Flow chart for bracketing procedure.

enough deficient skills to begin teaching the student. As an added check, the teacher tested Skill N. From the information obtained during the placement test, the teacher, parents, and possibly support personnel prioritize the skills to be taught that the student was not able to perform.

TABLE 2-II
TEACHING RESEARCH PLACEMENT TEST: GROSS MOTOR SKILLS

BRACKETING PROCEDURE

		Program and Suggested Cue	Placement Test				Baseline		Posttest		Comments
			Trial	Data	Yes/No	Date	Data	Date	Data	Date	
		GROSS MOTOR									
	A	Lifts head from teacher's shoulder – (physical cue)									
	B	Looks at light – (present light source)									
	C	Attends to face – (talk in stimulating way, using facial expression)									
I	D	Head extension on ball – (physical cue)									
	E	Lifts head while prone over bolster – (move stimulus upward in front of head)									
	F	Maintains head control when lifted – (physical cue)									
	G	Holds head in supported sitting – (physical cue)									
	H	Maintains head in midline –supine – (present stimulus at midline)	X X		Yes	9/28/78					
	I	Turns head – various positions – (present stimulus to the left and right sides alternately)	X Ⓞ Ⓧ		Yes	9/28/78					
	J	Bears weight on elbow when placed – (physical cue)	O X Ⓞ		No	9/28/78					
II	K	Rolls side to back – (move stimulus in direction of roll)	Ⓞ Ⓧ		Yes	9/28/78					
	L	Head righting on ball prone – (physical cue)	O O		No	9/28/78					
	M	Attains and maintains weight bearing on elbows – prone – (move stimulus upward in front of head)	O O		No	9/28/78					

Note: Each "physical cue" is individual to the program and refers to the placement and/or physical stimulation. See the sequences for specific information. A "stimulus" refers to any visual, auditory, or food stimulus that is interesting to the student, including adult's voice or face. Refer to the programs for suggestions.

Placement Testing

TABLE 2-II (continued)

	Program and Suggested Cue	Placement Test				Baseline		Posttest		Comments
		Trial	Data	Yes/No	Date	Data	Date	Data	Date	
	GROSS MOTOR (continued)									
N	Follows moving objects with eyes — (move stimulus in a complete circle in front of student and within five seconds)	O	/////	No	9/28/78					
O	Rolls from stomach to side — (move stimulus in direction of roll)	O	/////	No	9/28/78					
P	Bears weight on one elbow and reaches — prone — (place stimulus at arms reach in front of student)									
Q	Rolls from stomach to back — (move stimulus in direction of roll)									
R	Sits with support — (physical cue)									

REINFORCEMENT PROCEDURES

The procedures for reinforcement during a placement test, baseline test, and posttest are the same. Primary, tangible and/or social reinforcers *are* delivered throughout the placement test, contingent upon appropriate behaviors, such as attending to a task, maintaining eye contact, waiting patiently, following commands not related to the task being tested ("come here, sit down, give me the toy"), etc. Reinforcers are *not* delivered contingent upon correct performance on the specific test items. The rationale for this procedure is that delivery of reinforcers contingent upon correct performance constitutes treatment or teaching. On the other hand, the placement, baseline test (pretest), and posttests constitute evaluation of the student's performance prior to or after treatment. During these tests, however, reinforcers are delivered in order to maintain those behaviors (attention to task, sitting, waiting, etc.) necessary for a smooth and pleasant testing situation, and to keep the student motivated to continue attempting new tasks.

The frequency with which reinforcers are delivered is individual to each student. Profoundly handicapped students may require primary and social reinforcement at a high rate (every fifteen seconds), while the moderately handicapped adolescent may work for the entire placement test session given only periodic social praise and a free time break after thirty minutes as a reward. Again, the teacher can determine the frequency of reinforcement through information gathered from parents, from former teachers, and through her own informal observations prior to the placement test.

BASELINE. When placement is complete, the teacher, in conjunction with the parent and possibly support personnel, prioritizes skills that the student is lacking and chooses those skills to be taught. At this point a baseline is conducted to pinpoint specifically what phases and steps within each skill the student can or cannot perform. Thus, an accurate place to begin teaching a particular skill is determined. Because a student may have mastered portions of a skill before training begins, it is necessary to take a complete baseline. Begin baseline with the most difficult phase and/or step of the program and proceed to test easier phases or steps until the criterion of two out of two correct responses is obtained at any one phase or step. This will enable the teacher to skip teaching phases and steps the student knows. When baseline is completed, record the number of steps the student already has and the date on the placement test form (see Table 2-I).

POSTTEST. After a skill is completed, a posttest is given to be sure the behavior has been maintained in its entirety. Test the terminal objective only. Criterion is two out of two correct responses. When testing is completed successfully, record the date and total steps for the skill in the posttest column of the placement test and add to maintenance file if necessary. If testing is not completed successfully, probe the missed steps to determine where to begin teaching or to determine if the reinforcer needs to be faded more slowly. See the discussion of probing after a posttest.

PROBE. The baseline and posttest are conducted before and after a treatment program respectively; a probe is a test that is conducted primarily while the program is in progress. Pass criterion is two out of two correct responses, as for baseline and posttest procedures. Unlike the baseline, posttest, and placement tests, reinforcement *is* delivered for the target behavior being tested. There are four ways in which a probe can be utilized:

1. Review probe. A frequent and regular schedule of probes can be used to review the acquired skills in a multiple or noncumulative skill program.

2. Probe ahead. Students occasionally progress through programs at a much faster pace than we expect. This rapid progress usually occurs for one of two reasons: (1) the student was initially assessed erroneously in the program; (2) after the student has acquired the initial steps of a program, the remaining steps, which are extensions of the initial steps, are more easily acquired. A pattern of data indicating this phenomenon emerges when the student progresses through three to four steps with one or no errors; therefore, the decision of the teacher is to probe ahead. A probe of this nature presents a maximum of two trials, using the same reinforcers and schedule as during other programming.

3. Probe backward. When faced with data that reflect little or no success, there are certain considerations the teacher must make. There is the possibility that the poor performance of the student may be due to erroneous data at the previous step; therefore, the teacher should designate that the previous step be probed to ensure that the student is able to accomplish it. If the student can demonstrate in the probe that he can perform the previous step, the program probably needs to be branched (further breakdown of the task). If he cannot, he will have to be placed in the program where he can accomplish the step.

There may be a reason other than erroneous data for a student's being unable to perform the previous step of a program. The criterion level for moving to the next step may be set too low for mastery to occur, and the student may therefore "forget" the skill he learned on the previous day. If this phenomenon occurs more than once in a particular curricular area, the criterion for moving to the next step should be raised. For instance, if the criterion has been three consecutive responses before moving to the next step, it probably should be raised to five consecutive responses, possibly over two or more consecutive days.

4. Probe after posttest. If the student fails on the posttest, a probe of the

missed phases/steps can be conducted. This serves two purposes: (1) if the student was unsuccessful because he "forgot" how to perform the task, the teacher is able to identify where to begin reteaching; (2) since tangible/primary reinforcers are *not* delivered for correct performance of the target behavior during the posttest, failure on the posttest might indicate a need for the fading of the reinforcers used during the treatment program. Success on a probe conducted after an unsuccessful posttest would verify the need for a reinforcer fade (since reinforcers *are* delivered during the probe for correct performance).

Table 2-III

TEACHING RESEARCH PLACEMENT TEST

MOTOR SKILLS

	Program and Suggested Cue	Placement Test				Baseline			Posttest		Comments
		Trial	Data	Yes/No	Date	Data	Date		Data	Date	
	GROSS MOTOR										
A	Lifts head from teacher's shoulder – (physical cue)										
B	Looks at light – (present light source)										
C	Attends to face – (talk in stimulating way, using facial expression)										
D	Head extension on ball – (physical cue)										
E	Lifts head while prone over bolster – (move stimulus upward in front of head)										
F	Maintains head control when lifted – (physical cue)										
G	Holds head in supported sitting – (physical cue)										
H	Maintains head in midline – supine – (present stimulus at midline)										
I	Turns head – various positions – (present stimulus to the left and right sides alternately)										
J	Bears weight on elbows when placed – (physical cue)										
K	Rolls side to back – (move stimulus in direction of roll)										
L	Head righting on ball – prone – (physical cue)										
M	Attains and maintains weight bearing on elbows – prone – (move stimulus upward in front of head)										

Note: Each "physical cue" is individual to the program and refers to placement and/or physical stimulation. See the sequences for specific information. A "stimulus" refers to any visual, auditory, or food stimulus that is interesting to the student, including adult's voice or face. Refer to the programs for suggestions.

TEACHING RESEARCH PLACEMENT TEST
(continued)

Program and Suggested Cue	Placement Test				Baseline		Posttest		Comments
	Trial	Data	Yes/No	Date	Data	Date	Data	Date	
GROSS MOTOR *(continued)*									
N Follows moving objects with eyes – (move stimulus in a complete circle in front of student and within five seconds)		/////							
O Rolls from stomach to side – (move stimulus in direction of roll)		/////							
P Bears weight on one elbow and reaches – prone – (place stimulus at arms reach in front of student)		/////							
Q Rolls from stomach to back – (move stimulus in direction of roll)		/////							
R Sits with support – (physical cue)		/////							
S Bears weight on extended arms – sitting – (physical cue)		/////							
T Lifts head – supine – (present stimulus close to student's body just out of arms' reach)		/////							
U Rolls from back to side – (move stimulus in direction of roll)		/////							
V Bears weight on extended arms – prone (physical cue)		/////							
W Pulls to sit without head lag – (physical cue)		/////							
X Lifts head and shoulders – supine – (present stimulus close to student's body just out of arms' reach)		/////							
Y Pushes up on extended arms – prone – (move stimulus upward in front of head)		/////							
Z Protective extension forward on ball or bolster – (physical cue)		/////							
AA Protective extension – forward – (physical cue)		/////							
BB Rolls from side lying to stomach – (move stimulus in direction of roll)		/////							

Note: Each "physical cue" is individual to the program and refers to placement and/or physical stimulation. See the sequences for specific information. A "stimulus" refers to any visual, auditory, or food stimulus that is interesting to the student, including adult's voice or face. Refer to the programs for suggestions.

TEACHING RESEARCH PLACEMENT TEST
(continued)

	Program and Suggested Cue	Placement Test				Baseline		Posttest		Comments
		Trial	Data	Yes/No	Date	Data	Date	Data	Date	
	GROSS MOTOR *(continued)*									
CC	Rolls from back to stomach – (move stimulus in direction of roll)									
DD	Weight bearing with ball – (physical cue)									
EE	Sits without support – (physical cue)									
FF	Stands with support – (physical cue)									
GG	Pivots on stomach – (move stimulus to the side 180°)									
HH	Lifts adbomen in prone position – (move stimulus upward in front of head)									
II	Bears weight on hands and knees when placed – (physical cue)									
JJ	Bears weight on one extended arm and reaches – hands and knees – (present stimulus in front of student)									
KK	Moves toward an object – (present stimulus in front of student)									
LL	Moves forward down ramp – "Come." (present stimulus at other end of ramp)									
MM	Crawls forward on floor – "Come." (present stimulus at 5-foot distance)									
NN	Leans and regains balance, sitting position – (physical cue)									
OO	Protective extension – lateral – (physical cue)									
PP	Gets to sitting from prone – "Sit up." (move stimulus in direction of sitting movement)									
QQ	Gets to hands and knees – (physical cue)									

Note: Each "physical cue" is individual to the program and refers to placement and/or physical stimulation. See the sequences for specific information. A "stimulus" refers to any visual, auditory, or food stimulus that is interesting to the student, including adult's voice or face. Refer to the programs for suggestions.

TEACHING RESEARCH PLACEMENT TEST
(continued)

	Program and Suggested Cue	Trial	Placement Test Data	Placement Test Yes/No	Date	Baseline Data	Baseline Date	Posttest Data	Posttest Date	Comments
	GROSS MOTOR *(continued)*									
RR	Gets to sitting from hands and knees — "Sit." (move stimulus to the side)									
SS	Pulls to kneel stand — "Up." (present stimulus at support level)									
TT	Independent weight bearing — grasp — (physical cue)									
UU	Standing — no grasp ability — (physical cue)									
VV	Lifts trunk with hands and arms — (move stimulus upward in front of head)									
WW	Creeps on hands and knees — "Come." (present stimulus at 5-foot distance)									
XX	Turns trunk in sitting position — "Look." (present stimulus 6 foot from shoulder at side)									
YY	Gets to standing from hands and knees — "Stand up." (move stimulus upward)									
ZZ	Gets to sitting from supine — "Sit up." (move stimulus in appropriate direction)									
AAA	Creeps on hands and knees, negotiating environment — "Come." (move stimulus in appropriate direction)									
BBB	Cruises — "Come." (move stimulus in appropriate direction)									
CCC	Independent movement — grasp — "Come." (move stimulus in appropriate direction)									
DDD	Walking — no grasp ability — "Come." (move stimulus in appropriate direction)									
EEE	Gets to sitting from standing — "Sit." (present object on floor)									
FFF	Sits in chair — (physical cue)									

Note: Each "physical cue" is individual to the program and refers to placement and/or physical stimulation. See the sequences for specific information. A "stimulus" refers to any visual, auditory, or food stimulus that is interesting to the student, including adult's voice or face. Refer to the programs for suggestions.

TEACHING RESEARCH PLACEMENT TEST
(continued)

Program and Suggested Cue		Placement Test			Baseline		Posttest		Comments
		Trial	Data	Yes/No	Date	Data	Date	Data	Date	
	GROSS MOTOR *(continued)*									
GGG	Gets up from a chair – "Stand up."									
HHH	Falls forward – (physical cue)									
III	Gets into a chair – "Sit down."									
JJJ	Walks up incline – "Come." (present stimulus at 8-foot distance)									
KKK	Kneels – "Do this." (model)									
LLL	Bears weight on one knee – half-kneeling position – "Do this." (model)									
MMM	Creeps up steps – "Come."									
NNN	Rides on ride-on toy – "Come." – (place student on toy)									
OOO	Walks backward – "Do this." (model)									
PPP	Walks down incline – "Come." (present stimulus at 8-foot distance)									
QQQ	Creeps down stairs – "Come." (present stimulus five steps down)									
RRR	Walks up stairs – "Come."									
SSS	Walks down stairs – "Come."									
TTT	Picks up object from floor – standing – "Pick it up."									
UUU	Running – "Let's run." (run 300 yards with student)									
VVV	Seat self at table – "Sit down."									
WWW	Rides tricycle – "Come here."									
XXX	Jumps – "Do this." (model)									

Note: Each "physical cue" is individual to the program and refers to placement and/or physical stimulation. See the sequences for specific information. A "stimulus" refers to any visual, auditory, or food stimulus that is interesting to the student, including adult's voice or face. Refer to the programs for suggestions.

TEACHING RESEARCH PLACEMENT TEST
(continued)

Program and Suggested Cue		Placement Test			Baseline		Posttest		Comments
	Trial	Data	Yes/No	Date	Data	Date	Data	Date	
GROSS MOTOR *(continued)*									
YYY Stands on tiptoes with eyes open – "Do this." (model position)									
ZZZ Walks backward on a line – "Do this." (model)									
AAAA Stands on one foot, eyes open – "Do this." (model)									
BBBB Walks forward on a balance beam – "Do this." (model)									
CCCC Stands heel to toe – "Do this." (model)									
DDDD Stands on tiptoes, eyes closed – "Do this." (model position) "Close your eyes."									
EEEE Stands on one foot, eyes closed – "Do this." (model position) "Close your eyes."									
FINE MOTOR									
A Maintains grasp on object – supine – "Hold." (position object in hand and model)									
B Brings hands together – "Touch." (use any means to bring hands to midline and model)									
C Reaches for suspended swinging objects – supine – "Reach." (model)									
D Reaches for object – prone – "Reach." (model)									
E Reaches for and picks up, using whole hand grasp – "Pick it up." (model)									
F Grasps object with both hands – "Pick it up." (model)									
G Intentionally releases object from grasp – "Give it to me."									
H Transfers object from one hand to the other – "Put it here." (tap opposite palm)									

TEACHING RESEARCH PLACEMENT TEST
(continued)

	Program and Suggested Cue	Placement Test				Baseline			Posttest		Comments
		Trial	Data	Yes/No	Date	Data	Date		Data	Date	
	FINE MOTOR *(continued)*										
I	Grasps two objects, one in each hand – "Hold." (place small object in each hand and model)										
J	Reaches for and picks up object, using thumb/fingertips grasp – "Pick it up." (model)										
K	Picks up and grasps object, using neat pincer grasp (thumb and index finger) – "Pick it up." (model)										
L	Puts objects in small-mouthed container – "Put them in." (model)										
M	Moves object from one container to another – "Put it here." (tap empty container and model)										
N	Puts rings on a peg – "Put them on." (model)										
O	Builds a tower – "Stack the blocks." (model)										
P	Turns knob (specific to materials used. Example: "Open the door." "Turn it on."										
Q	Turns pages of a book, one at a time – "Turn the page." (model)										
R	Puts cylinders in same-sized receptable – "Put them in."										
S	Puts pegs in pegboard – "Put them in." (model)										
T	Strings beads – "String the beads." (model)										
U	Unscrews and screws on jar lid – "Open." (model)										
V	Pastes paper – "Paste it on." (model)										
W	Uses tongs to pick up objects – "Pick it up." (model)										
X	Cuts with scissors – "Cut out the circle; stay on the line." (model)										
Y	Laces ten-hole card – "Lace the circle." (model)										

Chapter 3

GROSS MOTOR SKILLS

THE MOTOR DEVELOPMENT section of the curriculum, like other sections, is organized in a developmental sequence. However, all students may not necessarily follow these same developmental sequences. A student may acquire skills in a different order. For example, some students will creep on their hands and knees before pulling to a standing position; others will pull to a standing position first before creeping on hands and knees. However, no student will deviate greatly from the developmental order of sequences; therefore, one cannot expect successful training at a later skill without a strong foundation of earlier acquired skills.

The developmental ages are provided only as guidelines to the teacher. These are the approximate ages at which the skill is acquired by a non-handicapped child. In addition, developmental ages for each program have some inherent difficulties. Some skills take two to eight months to acquire in a "normal" child's development. The program is placed in the curriculum at the time the earliest phase might be expected, but subsequent phases are labeled with the expected age for the development of that skill. Teachers should be very careful not to expect the student to move too rapidly through some of the programs. Thus, a student may be held at a particular phase and the program may be temporarily aborted for several months, with the teacher's probing occasionally to see if the student is ready for the next phase.

The teacher is referred to the *Data Based Classroom for the Moderately and Severely Handicapped* (Fredericks et al., 1979) for a data system that will allow her to determine whether or not the student should continue in the program if he is not succeeding. No student should continue in a program for which he is not ready and for which the data indicate that he is not succeeding over a period of time. Conversely, no student should be required to lockstep through a program if he is capable of moving ahead more rapidly. Again, the data will dictate that movement.

Some students, after they are given the idea of the skill that is desired, may be able to get closer to the program objective by using their own method of physical movement. If this occurs, the teacher should rewrite the program to incorporate the student's method, unless the student is using a pattern that can be harmfully abnormal. An example is "rolling over" using an extensor thrust movement to achieve the behavior.

TAXONOMY

The taxonomy for this chapter is divided into two sections. The first lists the skills in developmental order. The second lists those same skills, again in developmental order, but divided into categories of activities so that the teacher, therapist, and parent can ascertain the sequential order for these groups of skills such as sitting, forward movement (prone), and standing.

GLOSSARY

A glossary of terms relating to motor development, motion dysfunctions, and physical therapy is provided at the back of this volume.

REFERENCES

Fredericks, H. D., Baldwin, V. L., Moore, W., Piazza-Templeman, V., Grove, D., Moore, M., Gage, M. A., Blair, L., Alrick, G., Wadlow, M., Fruin, C., Bunse, C., Makohon, L., Samples, B., Moses, C., Rogers, G., Toews, J.: *A Data Based Classroom for the Moderately and Severely Handicapped,* 3rd ed. Monmouth, Instructional Development Corporation, 1979.

GROSS MOTOR SKILLS

Skill	Approximate Age for Skill Acquisition
A. Lifts Head from Teacher's Shoulder	1-3 months
B. Looks at Light	1-3 months
C. Attends to Face	1-2 months
D. Head Extension on Ball	1-4 months
E. Lifts Head while Prone over Bolster	1-3 months
F. Maintains Head Control when Lifted	1-5 months
G. Holds Head in Supported Sitting	2-3 months
H. Maintains Head in Midline — Supine	3 months
I. Turns Head — Various Positions	3-4 months
J. Bears Weight on Elbows when Placed	3-4 months
K. Rolls Side to Back	3-4 months
L. Head Righting on Ball — Prone	3-6 months
M. Attains and Maintains Weight Bearing on Elbows — Prone	3-4 months
N. Follows Moving Objects with Eyes	3-60 months
O. Rolls from Stomach to Side	4-5 months
P. Bears Weight on One Elbow and Reaches — Prone	4-6 months
Q. Rolls from Stomach to Back	4-6 months
R. Sits with Support	4-6 months
S. Bears Weight on Extended Arms — Sitting	5-6 months
T. Lifts Head — Supine	5-7 months

Gross Motor Skills

U.	Rolls from Back to Side	5-6 months
V.	Bears Weight on Extended Arms — Prone	5-7 months
W.	Pulls to Sit without Head Lag	6-8 months
X.	Lifts Head and Shoulders — Supine	6-9 months
Y.	Pushes Up on Extended Arms — Prone	6-7 months
Z.	Protective Extension Forward on Ball or Bolster	6-7 months
AA.	Protective Extension — Forward	6-8 months
BB.	Rolls from Side Lying to Stomach	7-8 months
CC.	Rolls from Back to Stomach	7-8 months
DD.	Weight Bearing with Ball	7-8 months
EE.	Sits without Support	7-8 months
FF.	Stands with Support	7-9 months
GG.	Pivots on Stomach	7-9 months
HH.	Lifts Abdomen in Prone Position	8-9 months
II.	Bears Weight on Hands and Knees when Placed	8-9 months
JJ.	Bears Weight on One Extended Arm and Reaches — Hands and Knees	8-10 months
KK.	Moves toward an Object	9-10 months
LL.	Moves Forward Down Ramp	9-10 months
MM.	Crawls Forward on Floor	9-10 months
NN.	Leans and Regains Balance, Sitting Position	9-10 months
OO.	Protective Extension — Lateral	9-10 months
PP.	Gets to Sitting from Prone	9-10 months
QQ.	Gets to Hands and Knees	9-10 months
RR.	Gets to Sitting from Hands and Knees	9-10 months
SS.	Pulls to Kneel Stand	9-11 months
TT.	Independent Weight Bearing — Grasp	9-12 months
UU.	Standing — No Grasp Ability	9-12 months
VV.	Lifts Trunk with Hands and Arms	9-12 months
WW.	Creeps on Hands and Knees	10-12 months
XX.	Turns Trunk in Sitting Position	10-12 months
YY.	Gets to Standing from Hands and Knees	10-16 months
ZZ.	Gets to Sitting from Supine	11-12 months
AAA.	Creeps on Hands and Knees, Negotiating Environment	10-14 months
BBB.	Cruises	10-14 months
CCC.	Independent Movement — Grasp	11-16 months
DDD.	Walking — No Grasp Ability	11-16 months
EEE.	Gets to Sitting from Standing	12-13 months
FFF.	Sits in Chair	12-16 months

GGG.	Gets Up from a Chair	12-16 months
HHH.	Falls Forward	13-16 months
III.	Gets into a Chair	13-20 months
JJJ.	Walks Up Incline	14-17 months
KKK.	Kneels	14-18 months
LLL.	Bears Weight on One Knee — Half-Kneeling Position	14-18 months
MMM.	Creeps Up Steps	15-17 months
NNN.	Rides on Ride-On Toy	15-20 months
OOO.	Walks Backward	16-18 months
PPP.	Walks Down Incline	16-18 months
QQQ.	Creeps Down Stairs	18-20 months
RRR.	Walks Up Stairs	18-36 months
SSS.	Walks Down Stairs	21-60 months
TTT.	Picks Up Object from Floor — Standing	21-30 months
UUU.	Running	2-4 years
VVV.	Seats Self at Table	2-3 years
WWW.	Rides Tricycle	2-4 years
XXX.	Jumps	3-5 years
YYY.	Stands on Tiptoes with Eyes Open	4-6 years
ZZZ.	Walks Backward on a Line	5-7 years
AAAA.	Stands on One Foot, Eyes Open	5-6 years
BBBB.	Walks Forward on a Balance Beam	5-6 years
CCCC.	Stands Heel to Toe	5-6 years
DDDD.	Stands on Tiptoes, Eyes Closed	5-7 years
EEEE.	Stands on One Foot, Eyes Closed	5-7 years

HEAD CONTROL

	Skill	Approximate Age for Skill Acquisition
A.	Lifts Head from Teacher's Shoulder	1-3 months
D.	Head Extension on Ball	1-4 months
E.	Lifts Head while Prone over Bolster	1-3 months
F.	Maintains Head Control when Lifted	1-5 months
G.	Holds Head in Supported Sitting	2-3 months
H.	Maintains Head in Midline — Supine	3 months
I.	Turns Head — Various Positions	3-4 months
L.	Head Righting on Ball — Prone	3-6 months
T.	Lifts Head — Supine	5-7 months
W.	Pulls to Sit without Head Lag	6-8 months
X.	Lifts Head and Shoulders — Supine	6-9 months

Gross Motor Skills

ROLLING

K.	Rolls Side to Back	3-4 months
O.	Rolls from Stomach to Side	4-5 months
Q.	Rolls from Stomach to Back	4-6 months
T.	Lifts Head — Supine	5-7 months
U.	Rolls from Back to Side	5-6 months
BB.	Rolls from Side Lying to Stomach	7-8 months
CC.	Rolls from Back to Stomach	7-8 months

TRACKING WITH EYES

B.	Looks at Light	1-3 months
C.	Attends to Face	1-2 months
N.	Follows Moving Objects with Eyes	3-60 months

SITTING

G.	Holds Head in Supported Sitting	2-3 months
R.	Sits with Support	4-6 months
S.	Bears Weight on Extended Arms — Sitting	5-6 months
EE.	Sits Without Support	7-9 months
NN.	Leans and Regains Balance, Sitting Position	9-10 months
OO.	Protective Extension — Lateral	9-10 months
PP.	Gets to Sitting from Prone	9-10 months
XX.	Turns Trunk in Sitting Position	10-12 months
FFF.	Sits in Chair	12-16 months

FORWARD MOVEMENT — PRONE

D.	Head Extension on Ball	1-4 months
J.	Bears Weight on Elbows when Placed	3-4 months
M.	Attains and Maintains Weight Bearing on Elbows — Prone	3-4 months
P.	Bears Weight on One Elbow and Reaches — Prone	4-6 months
V.	Bears Weight on Extended Arms — Prone	5-7 months
Y.	Pushes up on Extended Arms — Prone	6-7 months
GG.	Pivots on Stomach	7-9 months
KK.	Moves toward an Object	9-10 months
LL.	Moves Forward Down Ramp	9-10 months
MM.	Crawls Forward on Floor	9-10 months
WW.	Creeps on Hands and Knees	10-12 months
AAA.	Creeps on Hands and Knees, Negotiating Environment	10-14 months

Transitions

Q.	Rolls from Stomach to Back	4-6 months
CC.	Rolls from Back to Stomach	7-8 months
PP.	Gets to Sitting from Prone	9-10 months
QQ.	Gets to Hands and Knees	9-10 months
RR.	Gets to Sitting from Hands and Knees	9-10 months
SS.	Pulls to Kneel Stand	9-11 months
YY.	Gets to Standing from Hands and Knees	10-16 months
ZZ.	Gets to Sitting from Supine	11-12 months
EEE.	Gets to Sitting from Standing	12-13 months

Protective Extension

S.	Bears Weight on Extended Arms — Sitting	5-6 months
V.	Bears Weight on Extended Arms — Prone	5-7 months
Y.	Pushes Up on Extended Arms — Prone	6-7 months
Z.	Protective Extension Forward on Ball or Bolster	6-7 months
AA.	Protective Extension — Forward	6-8 months
II.	Bears Weight on Hands and Knees when Placed	8-9 months
JJ.	Bears Weight on One Extended Arm and Reaches — Hands and Knees	8-10 months
OO.	Protective Extension — Lateral	9-10 months
HHH.	Falls Forward	13-16 months

Hands and Knees

HH.	Lifts Abdomen in Prone Position	8-9 months
II.	Bears Weight on Hands and Knees when Placed	8-9 months
JJ.	Bears Weight on One Extended Arm and Reaches — Hands and Knees	8-10 months
QQ.	Gets to Hands and Knees	9-10 months
WW.	Creeps on Hands and Knees	10-12 months

Standing

DD.	Weight Bearing with Ball	7-8 months
FF.	Stands with Support	7-9 months
TT.	Independent Weight Bearing — Grasp	9-12 months
UU.	Standing — No Grasp Ability	9-12 months
YY.	Gets to Standing from Hands and Knees	10-16 months

Gross Motor Skills

WALKING OR RUNNING

BBB.	Cruises	10-14 months
CCC.	Independent Movement — Grasp	11-16 months
DDD.	Walking — No Grasp Ability	11-16 months
JJJ.	Walks Up Incline	14-17 months
OOO.	Walks Backward	16-18 months
PPP.	Walks Down Incline	16-18 months
UUU.	Running	24-48 months

STAIRS

MMM.	Creeps Up Stairs	15-17 months
QQQ.	Creeps Down Stairs	18-20 months
RRR.	Walks Up Stairs	18-36 months
SSS.	Walks Down Stairs	21-60 months

SUPPLEMENTAL ACTIVITIES

GGG.	Gets Up from a Chair	12-16 months
III.	Gets into a Chair	13-20 months
KKK.	Kneels	14-18 months
LLL.	Bears Weight on One Knee — Half-Kneeling Position	14-18 months
NNN.	Rides on Ride-On Toy	15-20 months
TTT.	Picks Up Object from Floor — Standing	21-30 months
VVV.	Seats Self at Table	2-3 years
WWW.	Rides Tricycle	2-4 years
XXX.	Jumps	3-5 years
YYY.	Stands on Tiptoes with Eyes Open	4-6 years
ZZZ.	Walks Backward on a Line	5-7 years
AAAA.	Stands on One Foot, Eyes Open	5-6 years
BBBB.	Walks Forward on a Balance Beam	5-6 years
CCCC.	Stands Heel to Toe	5-6 years
DDDD.	Stands on Tiptoes, Eyes Closed	5-7 years
EEEE.	Stands on One Foot, Eyes Closed	5-7 years

A. Lifts Head from Teacher's Shoulder

Approximate Age for
Skill Acquisition
1-3 months

TERMINAL OBJECTIVE: When held at teacher's shoulder, student will lift head and hold it steady for two minutes.

PREREQUISITE SKILLS: None.

Phase I — Place student at shoulder with free hand high on shoulders and back of neck. Teacher leans forward until student comes off shoulder, and she returns to upright. Student's head remains off shoulder. Pair with visual/auditory cue.

Phase II — Place student at shoulder with free hand high on shoulders and back of neck. Teacher leans forward until student lifts head briefly when gently rocked, bounced, or patted on back. Pair with visual/auditory cue.

Phase III — Place student at shoulder with free hand high on shoulders and back of neck. Teacher leans forward until student lifts head in response to visual/auditory cue. Teacher remains still.

Phase IV — Place student at shoulder with free hand high on shoulders and back of neck. Student lifts head in response to visual/auditory cue.

Phase V — Place student at shoulder with free hand high on shoulders and back of neck. Student lifts head independently.

The following steps are to be used with all of the phases:

Steps
1. Intermittent unsustained responses — lift and drop, lift and drop. Student extends neck and takes weight of head but holds only 2-5 seconds or perhaps momentarily then drops head to teacher's shoulder, rather than lowering carefully.
2. Two months. Student will sustain for thirty seconds.
3. Three months. Student will sustain for sixty seconds.
4. Three months. Student will sustain for ninety seconds.
5. Three months. Student will hold steady for 2 minutes.

SUGGESTED MATERIALS: Bright and/or moving object to use as visual/auditory cues. (Examples: red, squeaky ball; music box; rattle; or teacher's facial expressions.)

TEACHING NOTES:
1. Teaching Sequence — Teach Phase I, Step 1 and 2, then Phase II, Steps 1 and 2, continuing in the same manner through Phase V, Steps 1 and 2. At age of three months, teach Phase V, Steps 3, 4, and 5.
2. Note age norms for each step.
3. Visual/auditory cue may or may not elicit response in a normal one- to three-month-old student, but it is included for remediation purposes for the delayed student whose visual apparatus is physically more mature. In addition to the teacher's holding the student, another person may present the visual/auditory cue to elicit the head-holding behavior in the student.
4. *Caution:* This program requires modification by appropriate support personnel for use with students who have muscle tone problems, paralysis, or other physical handicaps.

B. Looks at Light

Approximate Age for
Skill Acquisition
1-3 months

TERMINAL OBJECTIVE:	Student looks at light source for three seconds, presented randomly within the field of vision.
PREREQUISITE SKILLS:	Ability to move eyes from side to side.
Phase I	Student looks at light source presented at eye level directly in front of face at a distance of approximately 15 to 20 inches.
Phase II	Student looks at light source presented at eye level directly to the left of student's face at a distance of approximately 15 to 20 inches.
Phase III	Student looks at light source presented at eye level directly to the right of student's face at a distance of approximately 15 to 20 inches.
Phase IV	Student looks at light source presented above eye level at a distance of approximately 15 to 20 inches.
Phase V	Student looks at light source presented below eye level at a distance of approximately 15 to 20 inches.
Phase VI	Student looks at light presented randomly within the field of vision at a distance of approximately 15 to 20 inches.

The following steps apply to Phases I through VI:

<u>Steps</u>

1. One second.
2. Two seconds.
3. Three seconds.

SUGGESTED MATERIALS:	Penlight or regular flashlight. Use alone or reflected off a shining or colorful object.
TEACHING NOTES:	1. Teaching Sequence — Teach this skill beginning with Phase I, Step 1. Then teach Phase I, Steps 2 and 3 before teaching Phase II, Steps 1 through 3. Continue to teach

remaining phases and steps in the same manner.
2. Position — Supine, reclined sitting.
3. It may be necessary when teaching this skill to use a dimly lit or semidark room. By doing so, the light source will be more visible.
4. "Field of vision" in Phase VI refers to the areas used in the previous phases — to the right, left, above, and below eye level.
5. In all phases light may be flashing or wiggling to get student's attention.
6. If student fails to make progress on this program, referral should be made for visual evaluation.
7. *Caution:* This program requires modification by appropriate support personnel for use with students who have muscle tone problems, paralysis, or other physical handicaps.

C. Attends to Face

Approximate Age for
Skill Acquisition
1-2 months

TERMINAL OBJECTIVE:	Student will attend to teacher's face for five seconds.
PREREQUISITE SKILLS:	None.
Phase I	With student fully supported directly in front of teacher, student attends to teacher's face when it is 12 inches from his.
Phase II	With student fully supported directly in front of teacher, student attends to teacher's face when it is 18 inches from his.

The following steps apply to both of the phases:

Steps

1. Two seconds.
2. Three seconds.
3. Four seconds.
4. Five seconds.

SUGGESTED MATERIALS: None.

TEACHING NOTES:
1. Teaching Sequence — Teach this skill beginning with Phase I, Step 1. Then teach Phase I, Steps 2 through 4 before teaching Phase II, Steps 1 through 4.
2. If student fails to make progress on this program, referral should be made for visual evaluation.
3. Teacher must make face interesting by expression and speaking.
4. *Caution:* This program requires modification by appropriate support personnel for use with students who have muscle tone problems, paralysis, or other physical handicaps.

D. Head Extension on Ball

Approximate Age for Skill Acquisition
1-4 months

Terminal Objective:	Student will, when placed in prone position on ball with arms in front of him raise head and push with arms to raise entire chest off ball. Student may extend arms.
Prerequisite Skills:	Lifts head at shoulder.
Phase I	One month. Student will, when placed in prone position on ball with arms flexed in front of him, raise face off ball far enough so that he can turn head. Turning head is OK but is not required.
Phase II	One to two months. Student will, when placed in prone position on ball with arms flexed in front of him, raise head off ball one-third of the way to 90° erect position (30° off ball).
Phase III	Two to three months. Student will, when placed in prone position on ball with arms flexed in front of him, raise head off ball two-thirds of the way to 90° erect position (60° off ball).
Phase IV	Three months. Student will, when placed in prone position on ball with arms flexed in front of him, raise head and push with arms to raise upper part of chest off ball.
Phase V	Four months. Student will, when placed in prone position on ball with arms flexed in front of him, raise head and push with arms to raise entire chest off ball. Student may extend arms.

The following steps are to be used with Phases II to V:

Steps
1. Two seconds.
2. Four seconds.
3. Six seconds.
4. Eight seconds.
5. Ten seconds.
6. Thirteen seconds.
7. Sixteen seconds.
8. Twenty seconds.
9. Twenty-five seconds.
10. Thirty seconds.

SUGGESTED MATERIALS: Large inflated ball, 36-inch size is the most versatile, but 4-foot size is also good. It should be used not fully inflated.

TEACHING NOTES:
1. Teaching Sequence — Teach this skill beginning with Phase I. Then teach Phase II, Steps 1 through 10 before teaching Phase III, Steps 1 through 10. Continue to teach all steps with each phase before going on to next phase.
2. Note age norms for each phase.
3. Gentle rocking or bouncing on ball may stimulate desired activity.
4. Very often a student may go up and down frequently rather than hold for the complete designated time. In those cases, the following set of steps, which are based on a percentage of a 30-second period, are appropriate and may be substituted for the steps listed previously:

    Steps

1. 10%	4. 40%	7. 70%	10. 100%
2. 20%	5. 50%	8. 80%	
3. 30%	6. 60%	9. 90%	

5. *Caution:* This program requires modification by appropriate support personnel for use with students who have muscle tone problems, paralysis, or other physical handicaps.

E. Lifts Head while Prone over Bolster

Approximate Age for Skill Acquisition
1-3 months

TERMINAL OBJECTIVE: When student is placed over bolster he will lift his head and hold it for thirty seconds.

PREREQUISITE SKILLS: Lifts head at shoulder.

Phase I — Student is placed in position on bolster. Gentle downward pressure is given over the hips with a slight rocking motion back and forth. With full physical assistance the student raises head and holds.

Phase II — Student is placed in position on bolster. Gentle downward pressure is given over the hips with a slight rocking motion back and forth. Teacher lifts student's head and releases it so that student is holding it upright intermittently. Teacher can lift student's head and release it repeatedly.

Phase III — Student is placed in position on bolster. Gentle downward pressure is given over the hips with a slight rocking motion back and forth. Teacher lifts student's head and releases it so that student is holding it upright intermittently. Teacher can lift student's head and release it repeatedly. Increase periods of non-support and stimulate extension by stroking fingers down either side of spine, patting bottom, as well as rocking or rolling bolster slightly forward.

Phase IV — Student is placed in position on bolster. Gentle downward pressure is given over the hips with a slight rocking motion back and forth. Teacher lifts student's head and releases it. Stimulate extension by stroking fingers down either side of spine, patting bottom, as well as rocking or rolling bolster slightly forward. Student holds head for prescribed time.

Phase V — Student is placed in position on bolster. Stimulate extension by stroking fingers down either side of spine, patting bottom, as well as rocking or rolling bolster slightly forward, and using auditory and visual cues. Student lifts head and holds it upright for prescribed time.

The following steps are to be used with Phases I through V:

Steps

1. Two seconds.
2. Five seconds.
3. Ten seconds.
4. Fifteen seconds.
5. Twenty seconds.
6. Twenty-five seconds.
7. Thirty seconds.

Phase VI Student is placed in position and lifts and holds head for thirty seconds in response to auditory and visual cues.

SUGGESTED MATERIALS:
1. Bolster: a long pillow or cushion wider than student's body. Firm, yet well-padded bolster. Diameter of bolster should be approximately the distance from student's armpit to elbow.
2. Bright and/or moving object to use as visual cue, e.g. mirror, mobile, wind chimes, music box.

TEACHING NOTES:
1. Teaching Sequence — Teach this skill beginning with Phase I, Step 1. Then teach Phase I, Steps 2 through 7 before teaching Phase II, Steps 1 through 7. Continue to teach remaining phases and steps in the same manner.
2. Use visual and auditory cues to stimulate head lifting.
3. Avoid pressure on throat. Bolster should be under chest with trunk, hips, and legs extended. At one month, hips and legs will not extend as much as they will at three months and later.
4. Very often a student may go up and down frequently, rather than hold for the complete designated time. In those cases, the

following set of steps, which are based on a percentage of a thirty-second time period, are appropriate and may be substituted for the steps listed previously.

<u>Steps</u>

1. 10%   4. 40%   7. 70%   10. 100%
2. 20%   5. 50%   8. 80%
3. 30%   6. 60%   9. 90%

5. *Caution:* This program requires modification by appropriate support personnel for use with students who have muscle tone problems, paralysis, or other physical handicaps.

F. Maintains Head Control when Lifted   Approximate Age for
                                               Skill Acquisition
                                               1-5 months

TERMINAL OBJECTIVE:	When student is lifted from a supine position, he supports his own head against gravity.
PREREQUISITE SKILLS:	Lifts head at shoulder.
Phase I	One month. Student will support his head against gravity when rolled to the side and lifted to teacher's shoulder. Teacher supports with hand under shoulders and head. Alternate sides.
Phase II	Student will support his head against gravity when rolled to the side and lifted to teacher's shoulder. Teacher supports with hand under shoulders and back of neck. Alternate sides.
Phase III	Two months. Student will support his head against gravity when rolled to the side and lifted to teacher's shoulders. Teacher supports with hand under shoulders. Alternate sides.
Phase IV	Three months. Student will support his head against gravity when rolled halfway to the side and lifted to teacher's shoulder. Teacher supports under shoulders and head. Alternate sides.
Phase V	Student will support his head against gravity when rolled halfway to the side and lifted to teacher's shoulder. Teacher supports under shoulders and back of neck. Alternate sides.
Phase VI	Student will support his head against gravity when rolled halfway to the side and lifted to teacher's shoulder. Teacher supports under shoulders. Alternate sides.
Phase VII	Student will support and lift his head against gravity when lifted straight up from supine. Teacher supports under shoulders and head.
Phase VIII	Four months. Student will support and lift head against gravity when lifted straight up from supine. Teacher supports under shoulders and back of neck.

Gross Motor Skills

Phase IX	Five months. Student will support and lift his head against gravity when lifted straight up from supine. Teacher supports under shoulders.
SUGGESTED MATERIALS:	Gym mat, foam pad, or bed to lie on.
TEACHING NOTES:	1. Teaching Sequence — Teach this skill beginning with Phase I. Then teach Phases II through IX.
2. Note age norms for each phase.
3. Data should be taken separately for left and right sides.
4. *Caution:* This program requires modification by appropriate support personnel for use with students who have muscle tone problems, paralysis, or other physical handicaps.

G. Holds Head in Supported Sitting

Approximate Age for Skill Acquisition
2-3 months

TERMINAL OBJECTIVE:	Student will hold head erect when supported around chest in sitting position for thirty seconds.
PREREQUISITE SKILLS:	Lifts head at shoulder and prone.
Phase I	Two months. Teacher holds student on lap, faced away, and leans child's back against her. Student's head does not drop forward.
Phase II	Teacher holds student on lap, facing teacher, and grasps one shoulder with each hand. Teacher assists student to hold head erect by moving shoulders.
Phase III	Three months. Teacher holds student on lap, facing teacher, and supports student with hands on each side of body under arms. Student holds head erect and steady.

The following steps apply to Phases I, II, and III:

Steps

1. Two seconds.
2. Three seconds.
3. Four seconds.
4. Five seconds.
5. Seven seconds.
6. Ten seconds.
7. Thirteen seconds.
8. Sixteen seconds.
9. Twenty seconds.
10. Twenty-five seconds.
11. Thirty seconds.

SUGGESTED MATERIALS: None.

TEACHING NOTES:
1. Teaching Sequence — Teach this skill beginning with Phase I, Steps 1 through 11. Then teach Phase II, Steps 1 through 11 before teaching Phase III, Steps 1 through 11.
2. Note age norms for Phases II and III.
3. *Caution:*
   a. This program requires modification by appropriate support personnel for use with students who have muscle tone

problems, paralysis, or other physical handicaps.
   b. Do not use Phase I with a cerebral palsied student.
4. Avoid having student tip head way back to look at teacher.

H. Maintains Head in Midline — Supine

Approximate Age for Skill Acquisition
3 months

TERMINAL OBJECTIVE: When student is lying supine he will maintain head at midline for ten seconds.

PREREQUISITE SKILLS: Turns head freely to both sides, beginning to support on forearms in prone position.

Phase I — On visual or auditory cue, teacher holds student's head in midline for ten seconds.

Phase II — On visual or auditory cue, teacher places student's head in midline and releases, reestablishing hold if student starts to turn to side.

The following steps are to be used with Phase II only:

Steps

1. Score correct if student makes any effort to hold. Score incorrect if the student turns immediately.
2. Two seconds.
3. Three seconds.
4. Four seconds.
5. Five seconds.
6. Six seconds.
7. Seven seconds.
8. Eight seconds.
9. Nine seconds.
10. Ten seconds.

Phase III — On visual or auditory cue student positions head at midline and maintains it.

The following steps are to be used with Phase III only.

Steps

1. Two seconds.
2. Three seconds.
3. Four seconds.
4. Five seconds.
5. Six seconds.
6. Seven seconds.
7. Eight seconds.
8. Nine seconds.
9. Ten seconds.

Gross Motor Skills

SUGGESTED MATERIALS:
1. Attention-getting toys, teacher's face to entertain.
2. Gym mat or foam pad to lie on.

TEACHING NOTES:
1. Teaching Sequence — Teach this skill beginning with Phase I. Then teach Phase II, Steps 1 through 10 before teaching Phase III, Steps 1 through 9.
2. Position — Student lying supine on floor, arms at side or hands together over chest or stomach. Legs extended between teacher's knees or flexed, resting in teacher's lap. Position of arms and legs should be symmetrical. Teacher must be midline to the student.
3. The term "midline" as used in this sequence requires the student to look straight up toward the ceiling.
4. Be certain that there are no distractors on either side and that the student has something to attend to at the midline, i.e. teacher's face.
5. *Caution:* This program requires modification by appropriate support personnel for use with students who have muscle tone problems, paralysis, or other physical handicaps.

I. Turns Head — Various Positions

Approximate Age for Skill Acquisition
3-4 months

TERMINAL OBJECTIVE: Student turns head in either direction (left and right) responding within two seconds to a sensory stimulus.

PREREQUISITE SKILLS: Ability to turn head left and right.

Phase I — Student turns head from midline in specified direction, responding within twenty seconds when presented with a sensory stimulus and complete physical assistance by teacher to turn head.

Phase II — Student turns head from midline in specified direction, responding within twenty seconds when presented with a sensory stimulus and physical assistance by teacher who touches head to initiate movement. Student follows through with movement.

Phase III — Student turns head from midline in specified direction, responding within twenty seconds when presented with a sensory stimulus.

Phase IV — Student turns head from midline in specified direction, responding within fifteen seconds when presented with a sensory stimulus.

Phase V — Student turns head from midline in specified direction, responding within ten seconds when presented with a sensory stimulus.

Phase VI — Student turns head from midline in specified direction, responding within five seconds when presented with sensory stimulus.

Phase VII — Student turns head from midline in specified direction, responding within two seconds when presented with a sensory stimulus.

The following steps are to be used with Phases I through VII:

<u>Steps</u>

1. Student turns head toward sensory stimulus to the left.
2. Student turns head toward sensory stimulus to the right.

SUGGESTED MATERIALS:
1. Toy or object to be used as sensory stimulus. Item should be selected on the basis of corresponding to the student's strongest sense or on the basis of what is most reinforcing to the student. Noise makers, bells, lights are some suggested items.
2. Gym mat, padded wedge, or supportive chair (see Teaching Note #2).

TEACHING NOTES:
1. Teaching Sequence — Teach this skill beginning with Phase I, teaching both Steps 1 and 2 in a single session. Then continue with Phases II through VII, always teaching both steps in a given training session.
2. Position can make a difference. Supine may be easiest or have the student sitting or reclined on a padded wedge, depending on student. Work this program first in the position where head turn is easiest for student. Then progress to other positions.
3. *Caution:* This program requires modification by appropriate support personnel for use with students who have muscle tone problems, paralysis, or other physical handicaps.

J. Bears Weight on Elbows when Placed

Approximate Age for
Skip Acquisition
3-4 months

TERMINAL OBJECTIVE:	Student bears weight on both elbows for thirty seconds when placed in a prone position.
PREREQUISITE SKILLS:	Lifts head over bolster and from teacher's shoulder.
Phase I	When placed in a prone position, student bears weight on both elbows with complete physical assistance.
Phase II	Student bears weight on both elbows when placed in a prone position with teacher supporting sides of arms, helping student to maintain position by tapping under chin gently.
Phase III	Student bears weight on both elbows when placed in a prone position with teacher supporting sides of arms when necessary to help. Student maintains position.
Phase IV	Student bears weight on both elbows when placed in a prone position with teacher lightly touching sides of arms, then releasing immediately. Student maintains position.
Phase V	Student bears weight on both elbows when placed in a prone position.

The following steps apply to Phases I through V:

Steps

1. Five seconds.
2. Ten seconds.
3. Fifteen seconds.
4. Twenty seconds.
5. Twenty-five seconds.
6. Thirty seconds.

SUGGESTED MATERIALS:
1. Interesting toys or mirror for student to look at may increase success.
2. Gym mat or padded carpet to lie on.

TEACHING NOTES:
1. Teaching Sequence — Teach this skill beginning with Phase I, Step 1. Then teach Phase I, Steps 2 through 6 before teaching Phase II, Steps 1 through 6. Continue to teach the remaining phases in the same manner.
2. *Caution:* This program requires modification by appropriate support personnel for use with students who have muscle tone problems, paralysis, or other physical handicaps.

K. Rolls Side to Back

Approximate Age for Skill Acquisition
3-4 months

TERMINAL OBJECTIVE: Student turns from side lying to supine by turning his face toward ceiling and reaching back with top arm. (In small baby, turning of head only may be sufficient.)

PREREQUISITE SKILLS: Turns head freely.

Phase I — Teacher assists student to turn head in appropriate direction by holding *gently* above the ears and turning *gently*. Visual/auditory cue positioned behind student or moving in direction of turn so student will follow.

Phase II — Teacher assists head turn with intermittent tapping (gentle pushing), turning face toward ceiling and tapping arm back. Visual or auditory cue positioned behind student or moving in direction of turn so student will follow.

Phase III — Teacher assists head turn with intermittent tapping (gentle pushing), turning face toward ceiling. Visual or auditory cue positioned behind student or moving in direction of turn so student will follow.

Phase IV — Student rolls side to back, seeking visual or auditory cue. Visual or auditory cue positioned behind student or moving in direction of turn so student will follow.

The following steps apply to Phases I through IV:

Steps
1. Rolls to left side.
2. Rolls to right side.

SUGGESTED MATERIALS:
1. Items that can be used as visual or auditory cues: bell, musical or noise toy, light, food, toys that are *both* visually and auditorily stimulating, voice of teacher.
2. Gym mat or padded carpet.

TEACHING NOTES:
1. Teaching Sequence — Teach this skill beginning with Phase I, teaching both steps in each training session. Then teach Phases II through IV in the same manner.
2. *Caution:* This program requires modification by appropriate support personnel for use with students who have muscle tone problems, paralysis, or other physical handicaps.

L. Head Righting on Ball — Prone

Approximate Age for Skill Acquisition
3-6 months

TERMINAL OBJECTIVE: When ball is tipped, student will turn face toward high side of ball.

PREREQUISITE SKILLS: Lifts head from teacher's shoulder and prone, prop on forearms must be beginning.

Phase I
Position. Student is placed on ball prone and rolled forward to a 45° head down position. Arms are forward along side of head.

The ball is then rolled to the right 30° or 40°. Student turns face to high side of ball (left). Teacher lifts student's left shoulder to assist. Repeat to opposite side.

Phase II
Position. Student is placed on ball in prone position and rolled forward to a 45° head down position. Arms are forward along side of head.

The ball is then rolled to the right 30° or 40°. Student turns face to high side of ball (left). Repeat for opposite side.

Phase III
Position. Student is placed prone on ball in horizontal position. Arms are forward along side of head.

Ball is rolled right 30° or 40°. Student turns face to high side of ball (left). Repeat to opposite side.

Phase IV
Position. Student is placed prone on ball in horizontal position. Arms are forward along side of head.

Ball is rolled right 30° or 40°. Student turns face to high side (left). Repeat to opposite side.

The following steps apply to Phases I through IV:

<u>Steps</u>

Student turns head —
1. within six seconds.
2. within four seconds.
3. within two seconds.
4. as ball moves.

SUGGESTED MATERIALS:	Large inflated beach ball with a 36- to 48-inch diameter.
TEACHING NOTES:	1. Teaching Sequence — Teach this skill beginning with Phase I, Steps 1 through 4. Then teach Phase II, Steps 1 through 4. Teach subsequent phases and steps in the same manner. 2. Bouncing student on ball may help stimulate and activate desired reactions prior to the teaching of this program. 3. *Caution:* This program requires modification by appropriate support personnel for use with students who have muscle tone problems, paralysis, or other physical handicaps.

M. Attains and Maintains Weight Bearing on Elbows — Prone

Approximate Age for Skill Acquisition
3-4 months

TERMINAL OBJECTIVE: Student raises head and props upper trunk on elbows while in prone position, maintaining position for ten seconds.

PREREQUISITE SKILLS: Student can bear weight on elbows when placed.

Phase I — In a prone position, student lifts head and shoulders off floor and props upper trunk on elbows and forearms, given complete physical assistance by teacher.

Phase II — In a prone position, student lifts head and shoulders off floor and props upper trunk on elbows and forearms, given physical assistance by teacher supporting student's shoulders.

Phase III — In a prone position, student lifts head and shoulders off floor and props upper trunk on elbows and forearms, given physical assistance by teacher supporting under chin.

Phase IV — In a prone position, student lifts head and shoulders off floor and props upper trunk on forearms and elbows.

The following steps apply to Phases I through IV:

Steps
1. Maintains position for two seconds.
2. Maintains position for four seconds.
3. Maintains position for six seconds.
4. Maintains position for eight seconds.
5. Maintains position for ten seconds.

SUGGESTED MATERIALS:
1. Visual/auditory cues can be used, especially in Phase IV.
2. Gym mat or padded carpet.

TEACHING NOTES:
1. Teaching Sequence — Teach this skill beginning with Phase I, Step 1. Then teach Phase I, Steps 2 through 5 before teaching Phase II, Steps 1 through 5. Continue to

teach remaining phases and steps in the same manner.
2. *Catuion:* This program requires modification by appropriate support personnel for use with students who have muscle tone problems, paralysis, or other physical handicaps.

N. Follows Moving Objects with Eyes

Approximate Age for
Skill Acquisition
3-60 months

TERMINAL OBJECTIVE: Student follows a moving object with eyes when object is moved in a complete 360° circle.

PREREQUISITE SKILLS: Ability to move eyes from left to right; ability to look at an object steadily.

Phase I — Three months. Student will follow a moving object with eyes 90° when moved horizontally from side to midline.

Phase II — Four months. Student will follow a moving object with eyes 180° when moved horizontally from side to side.

Phase III — Thirty-four months. Student will follow a moving object with eyes 90° when moved vertically from top of field of vision to midline.

Phase IV — Forty-eight months. Student will follow a moving object with eyes 180° when moved vertically from top of field of vision to bottom.

Phase V — Student will follow a moving object with eyes 90° when moved angularly from side to midline.

The following steps are to be used with Phase V:

Steps

1. Move from upper right to midline.
2. Move from upper left to midline.
3. Move from lower right to midline.
4. Move from lower left to midline.

Phase VI — Student will follow a moving object with eyes 180° when moved angularly from side to side.

The following steps are to be used with Phase VI:

Steps

1. Move from upper right to lower left.
2. Move from upper left to lower right.

3. Move from lower right to upper left.
4. Move from lower left to upper right.

Phase VII Thirty-four months. Student will follow a moving object with eyes in a 90° arc.

Phase VIII Thirty-four months. Student will follow a moving object with eyes in a 180° arc.

Phase IX Student will follow a moving object with eyes in a 270° arc.

Phase X Sixty months. Student will follow a moving object with eyes when moved in a complete 360° circle.

The following substeps are to be used with Phases I through X:

Substeps

a. Supported in sitting position, object moved slowly within a ten-second time period.
b. Supine position, object moved slowly within a ten-second time period.
c. Prone position, object moved slowly within a ten-second time period.
d. Supported in sitting position, object moved quickly within a five-second time period.
e. Supine position, object moved quickly within a five-second time period.
f. Prone position, object moved quickly within a five-second time period.

SUGGESTED MATERIALS:
1. Light- or bright-colored toy. Variety may be necessary within a given teaching session.
2. Gym mat or padded carpet.

TEACHING NOTES:
1. Teaching Sequence — Teach this skill beginning with Phase I, Step 1, Substeps a through f. Then teach Phase I, Step 2, substeps a through f. Teach subsequent steps of Phase I in the same manner. Teach all subsequent phases, steps, and substeps in the same manner.

2. Object is held in front of student at a distance of approximately 12 to 18 inches in front of eyes. For Phases VII through X the object is moved in a circular or arc pattern in front of the student.
3. Note age norms for each phase.
4. The teacher should use the position that is easiest for the student initially. Thus, the sequence of positions may vary from student to student, and the substeps listed may be presented in a different order.
5. If it becomes apparent that it is easier for the student to follow from midline to side as opposed to from side to midline, change sequence accordingly.
6. *Caution:* This program requires modification by appropriate support personnel for use with students who have muscle tone problems, paralysis, or other physical handicaps.

Gross Motor Skills 77

O. Rolls from Stomach to Side

Approximate Age for
Skill Acquisition
4-5 months

TERMINAL OBJECTIVE: With visual or auditory cue, student rolls from stomach to side.

PREREQUISITE SKILLS: Props on elbows and lifts head prone.

Phase I   Student props on elbows with head up independently. Teacher provides complete assistance for student to shift weight and turn head. Visual or auditory cue is moved in direction of turn so student will follow. Repeat for opposite side.

Phase II Student props on elbows with head up independently. Teacher taps shoulder to assist rolling. Visual or auditory cue moved in direction of turn so student will follow. Repeat for opposite side.

Phase III Student props on elbows with head up independently. Teacher uses visual or auditory cue to guide movement as student rolls from stomach to side. Repeat for opposite side.

SUGGESTED MATERIALS:
1. Things that can be used as visual or auditory cues: bell, musical or noise toy, light, food, toys that are *both* visually and auditorily stimulating, voice of teacher.
2. Gym mat or padded carpet.

TEACHING NOTES:
1. Teaching Sequence — Teach this skill beginning with Phase I, then teach Phase II before teaching Phase III. Student must work on rolling to both right and left in each training session.
2. This skill requires the student to begin in a prone position propped on elbows with head up to shift weight to one side, lower shoulder to mat. Task is complete when hips are in line with shoulders in side lying. *It is acceptable if student continues full roll to back lying but not required for this program.* Do not stop him from completing roll.

3. A sudden weight shift may elicit equilibrium reaction that will block the roll.
4. *Caution:* This program requires modification by appropriate support personnel for use with students who have muscle tone problems, paralysis, or other physical handicaps.

P. Bears Weight on One Elbow and Reaches — Prone

Approximate Age for Skill Acquisition
4-6 months

TERMINAL OBJECTIVE: Student in prone position bears weight on one elbow while reaching for and touching toy with free arm.

PREREQUISITE SKILLS: Props on elbows, turns head freely prone, reaches upward in supine.

Phase I With student propped on elbows, teacher holds (stabilizes) hips and assists weight shift to one elbow. (Student does not have to reach out with free arm for a correct response, but do not stop him if he does so.) Teacher holds shoulders to maintain shift.

Phase II With student propped on elbows, teacher stabilizes hips and assists weight shift to one elbow. (Student does not have to reach out with free arm for a correct response, but do not stop him if he does so.) Student maintains weight shift for designated time.

Phase III With student propped on elbows, teacher stabilizes hips and taps student to prompt shift to one elbow. (Student does not have to reach out with free arm for a correct response, but do not stop him if he does so.) Student maintains weight shift for designated time.

Phase IV With student propped on elbows, teacher taps student to prompt shift to one elbow. (Student does not have to reach out with free arm for a correct response, but do not stop him if he does so.) Student maintains weight shift for designated time.

The following steps are to be used with Phases I through IV:

<u>Steps</u>
1. One second.
2. Two seconds.
3. Three seconds.

Phase V	With student propped on elbows, teacher taps student to prompt shift to one elbow. Teacher then physically assists student to reach out and touch toy.
Phase VI	With student propped on elbows, teacher taps student to prompt shift to one elbow. Teacher then taps student's arm to prompt him to reach out and touch toy.
Phase VII	With student propped on elbows, student shifts to one elbow and reaches out and touches toy.

SUGGESTED MATERIALS:
1. Bright or noisy toys, music box, coffee can, small toys, or blocks.
2. Gym mat or padded carpet.

TEACHING NOTES:
1. Teaching Sequence — Teach Phase I, Steps 1, 2, and 3 before teaching Phase II, Steps 1, 2, and 3. Continue with Phases III and IV in the same manner and then teach Phases V, VI, and VII.
2. Teach this skill on both right and left sides each training session. Data should be maintained for each side.
3. *Caution:* This program requires modification by appropriate support personnel for use with students who have muscle tone problems, paralysis, or other physical handicaps.

Gross Motor Skills

Q. Rolls from Stomach to Back

Approximate Age for Skill Acquisition
4-6 months

TERMINAL OBJECTIVE:	Student will roll from stomach to back.
PREREQUISITE SKILLS:	Prop on elbows and turn head freely, shifts weight on elbows, rolls from stomach to side.
Phase I	Teacher, using auditory and visual cue, provides full assistance to shift weight, turn head, and complete move.
Phase II	Teacher, using auditory and visual cue, taps gently at shoulder, head, and hips if necessary to assist movement.
Phase III	With teacher using auditory/visual cue to guide movement, student rolls stomach to back.
SUGGESTED MATERIALS:	1. Attention-getting toys, music box, teacher's face. 2. Gym mat or padded carpet.
TEACHING NOTES:	1. Teaching Sequence — Teach Phase I, followed by Phases II and III. 2. Alternate sides to which the student rolls. If student rolls to side but cannot roll onto back because head is extended too far back, contact physical therapist. 3. This task is performed as follows: Student, propped and supported by elbows while lying on stomach with head up, shifts weight to one side and lowers shoulder to mat turning face toward ceiling and then on back in direction of roll. Movement complete when student's hips and shoulders are flat on mat in back lying. 4. *Caution:* This program requires modification by appropriate support personnel for use with students who have muscle tone problems, paralysis, or other physical handicaps.

R. Sits with Support

Approximate Age for
Skill Acquisition
4-6 months

TERMINAL OBJECTIVE: Student sits upright for thirty seconds, hands free, perpendicular to floor when given support at hips by teacher.

PREREQUISITE SKILLS: Lifts head prone, bears weight on elbows.

Phase I — Student sits upright, teacher supporting entire trunk, hips, and thighs in perpendicular position.

Phase II — Student sits upright, teacher supporting entire trunk and hips in position.

Phase III — Student sits upright, teacher supporting entire trunk, waist to shoulders.

Phase IV — Student sits upright, teacher supporting trunk around ribs.

Phase V — Student sits upright, teacher supporting waist.

Phase VI — Student sits upright, teacher supporting hips.

The following steps apply to all of the phases:

Steps

1. Five seconds.
2. Ten seconds.
3. Fifteen seconds.
4. Twenty seconds.
5. Twenty-five seconds.
6. Thirty seconds.

SUGGESTED MATERIALS: See Teaching Note #2.

TEACHING NOTES:
1. Teaching Sequence — Teach this skill beginning with Phase I, Step 1. Then teach Phase I, Steps 2 through 6 before teaching Phase II, Steps 1 through 6. Continue to teach the remaining phases and steps in the same manner.
2. This particular skill can be taught using a solid flat surface (floor, tabletop, etc.) or on teacher's lap.

3. *Caution:* This program requires modification by appropriate support personnel for use with students who have muscle tone problems, paralysis, or other physical handicaps.

S. Bears Weight on Extended Arms — Sitting

Approximate Age for Skill Acquisition
5-6 months

TERMINAL OBJECTIVE: Student bears weight on palms of hands for sixty seconds with elbows straight, while in an upright sitting position. Hands are placed between student's legs, which are extended in front of student.

PREREQUISITE SKILLS: Sits with support.

Phase I — Student bears weight on palms of hands with elbows straight while in an upright position, given complete physical assistance. Teacher holds elbows straight and palms flat on the surface.

Phase II — Student bears weight on palms of hands with elbows straight while in an upright position with complete physical assistance to hold elbows straight. Student keeps palms flat on surface.

Phase III — Student bears weight on palms of hands with elbows straight while in an upright position. Teacher positions student and continues touching elbows. Student maintains weight-bearing position.

Phase IV — Student bears weight on palms of hands with elbows straight while in an upright sitting position. Teacher positions elbows. Student maintains weight-bearing position independently.

Phase V — Student bears weight on palms of hands with elbows straight while in an upright sitting position.

The following steps are to be used with Phases I through V:

Steps

1. Five seconds.
2. Ten seconds.
3. Fifteen seconds.
4. Twenty seconds.

5. Twenty-five seconds.
6. Thirty seconds.
7. Sixty seconds.

SUGGESTED MATERIALS: None.

TEACHING NOTES:
1. Teaching Sequence — Teach Phase I, Steps 1 through 7 before teaching Phase II, Steps 1 through 7. Teach remaining phases in same manner.
2. *Caution:* This program requires modification by appropriate support personnel for use with students who have muscle tone problems, paralysis or other physical handicaps.

T. Lifts Head — Supine

Approximate Age for
Skill Acquisition
5-7 months

TERMINAL OBJECTIVE:	Lying supine, student will raise head 3 inches off floor.
PREREQUISITE SKILLS:	Maintain head in midline while in supine position.
Phase I	With student reclined against an incline of 45°, student lifts head 3 inches with full physical assistance from teacher.
Phase II	With student reclined against an incline of 45°, student lifts head 3 inches with teacher tapping head forward to assist.
Phase III	With student reclined against an incline of 45°, student lifts head 3 inches without help.
Phase IV	With student reclined against an incline of 30°, student lifts head 3 inches with full physical assistance from teacher.
Phase V	With student reclined against an incline of 30°, student lifts head 3 inches with teacher tapping head forward to assist.
Phase VI	With student reclined against an incline of 30°, student lifts head 3 inches without help.
Phase VII	With student reclined against an incline of 10°, student lifts head 3 inches with full physical assistance from teacher.
Phase VIII	With student reclined against an incline of 10°, student lifts head 3 inches with teacher tapping head forward to assist.
Phase IX	With student reclined against an incline of 10°, student lifts head 3 inches without help.
Phase X	With student lying supine on floor, student lifts head 3 inches with full physical assistance from teacher.
Phase XI	With student lying supine on floor, student lifts head 3 inches with teacher tapping head forward to assist.

Gross Motor Skills

Phase XII	With student lying supine on floor, student lifts head 3 inches without help.
SUGGESTED MATERIALS:	Attention-getting toys or pictures. Foam wedge or pillows for desired incline.
TEACHING NOTES:	1. Teaching Sequence — Teach this skill beginning with Phase I, then teach Phases II, III, IV, etc. 2. Suspend an object in front of the student so that when he raises his head he touches it with his nose or forehead. This in itself may be reinforcing or use tangible rewards. 3. *Caution:* This program requires modification by appropriate support personnel for use with students who have muscle tone problems, paralysis, or other physical handicaps.

U. Rolls from Back to Side

Approximate Age for
Skill Acquisition
5-6 months

TERMINAL OBJECTIVE:	Student, from a supine position, lifts head and turns face toward direction he is going to turn. Top arm reaches in direction of turn; shoulders and hips follow until student is lying on side.
PREREQUISITE SKILLS:	Lifts head supine, turns head freely, hands cross midline.
Phase I	Teacher provides complete assistance for student to lift head, turn face, and bring top shoulder and arm forward. Visual or auditory item is moved in direction of turn for student to look at and reach for it. Repeat for opposite side.
Phase II	Teacher taps student's head and shoulder to initiate roll; student completes roll to side. Visual or auditory item is moved in direction of turn for student to look at and reach for it. Repeat for opposite side.
Phase III	Teacher taps student's head to initiate roll. Student completes roll to side. Visual or auditory item is moved in direction of turn for student to look at and reach for it. Repeat for opposite side.
Phase IV	Student completes roll independently. Visual or auditory item is moved in direction of turn for student to look at and reach for it. Repeat for opposite side.
SUGGESTED MATERIALS:	1. Items that can be used as visual or auditory cues: bells, musical or noise toys, light, food, toys that are *both* visually and auditorily stimulating, voice of trainer. 2. Gym mat or padded carpet.
TEACHING NOTES:	1. Teaching Sequence — Begin teaching this skill with Phase I. Then teach Phases II, III, and IV.

2. A verbal cue can be used. This sequence might be, "Roll over; get the toy."
3. Work to both right and left during each training session. Separate data should be taken for each side.
4. Phases I and II may be started before student is lifting head in supine position.
5. *Do not restrict student if he continues to roll to stomach,* but this is not required for this skill.
6. *Caution:* This program requires modification by appropriate support personnel for use with students who have muscle tone problems, paralysis, or other physical handicaps.

V. Bears Weight on Extended Arms — Prone

Approximate Age for Skill Acquisition
5-7 months

TERMINAL OBJECTIVE: Student will sustain weight of upper trunk on extended arms for thirty seconds.

PREREQUISITE SKILLS: Bears weight on elbows, prone; bears weight on extended arms, sitting.

Phase I   With student in prone position and palms of hands on flat surface, teacher lifts student with shoulders and bounces gently on hands. Student pushes briefly against surface.

(Alternate) With student across teacher's lap in full extension of hips and spine, teacher lifts student gently under chin. Teacher is sitting on floor. Student pushes up and rests weight on hands.

(Alternate) Student lies prone over large bolster and is pushed forward until weight rests on hands.

Phase II   With student in prone position, teacher assists student to assume weight-bearing position. Teacher encourages student to hold by tapping gently under chin or chest.

Phase III   Student is assisted to weight-bearing position and sustains it.

The following steps are to be used with Phases II and III only:

Steps
1. Two seconds.
2. Three seconds.
3. Four seconds.   } 5 months
4. Five seconds.
5. Ten seconds.
6. Fifteen seconds.
7. Twenty seconds.   } 6 months
8. Twenty-five seconds.
9. Thirty seconds.   7 months

SUGGESTED MATERIALS: Firm, yet well-padded bolster (for alternate to

Gross Motor Skills

Phase I). Diameter of bolster should be approximately the distance from student's armpit to hand.

TEACHING NOTES:
1. Teaching Sequence — Teach this skill beginning with Phase I. Then teach Phase II, Steps 1 through 9, before teaching Phase III, Steps 1 through 9.
2. Very often a student may go up and down frequently rather than hold for the complete designated time. In those cases, the following set of steps, which are based on a percentage of a thirty-second period, are appropriate and may be substituted for the steps listed previously:

Steps
1. 10%   4. 40%   7. 70%   10. 100%
2. 20%   5. 50%   8. 80%
3. 30%   6. 60%   9. 90%

3. *Caution:* This sequence requires modification by appropriate support personnel for use with students who have muscle tone problems, paralysis, or other physical handicaps.

W. Pulls to Sit without Head Lag

Approximate Age for
Skill Acquisition
6-8 months

TERMINAL OBJECTIVE:	Student will maintain head control when pulled to a sitting position by hands.
PREREQUISITE SKILLS:	Maintains head control when lifted.
Phase I	Given support at head, neck, and shoulders (shoulders rolled forward), student will maintain head control when pulled to a sitting position.
Phase II	Given support at neck and shoulders (shoulders rolled forward), student will maintain head control when pulled to a sitting position.
Phase III	Given support at shoulders (shoulders rolled forward) student will maintain head control when pulled to a sitting position.
Phase IV	Student will maintain head control when pulled to a sitting position by hands.

The following steps apply to Phases I through IV:

Steps

1. Lifted up from an inclined board 60° from floor.
2. Lifted up from an inclined board 45° from floor.
3. Lifted up from an inclined board 30° from floor.
4. Lifted up from floor.

SUGGESTED MATERIALS: Padded incline board or foam wedge; attention-getting toys.

TEACHING NOTES:
1. Teaching Sequence — Teach this skill beginning with Phase I, Step 1. Then teach Phase I, Steps 2 through 4 before teaching Phase II, Steps 1 through 4. Continue to teach remaining phases and steps in the same manner.
2. If student is unable to accomplish this skill, it may be taught in reverse; the student will hold head forward against gravity while lowering from sitting to supine. Teacher

holds shoulders forward. Steps 1 through 4 the same. Once the reverse has been taught, the skill may be taught as listed.
3. When pulling the student (especially the infant) up to sitting by the arms, begin by tugging gently until you feel him resist pull with his arms before continuing to pull. This will avoid injury to shoulder joints.
4. *Caution:* This program requires modification by appropriate support personnel for use with students who have muscle tone problems, paralysis, or other physical handicaps.

X. Lifts Head and Shoulders — Supine

Approximate Age for Skill Acquisition
6-9 months

TERMINAL OBJECTIVE:	Lying supine, student lifts head and shoulders up enough so teacher can slide hand under shoulder blades without resistance.
PREREQUISITE SKILLS:	No head lag when pulled to sit; lifts head supine.
Phase I	Student is seated, reclined against an incline of 45°. Student lifts head and teacher assists lifting of shoulders.
Phase II	Student is seated, reclined against an incline of 45°. Student lifts head and shoulders.
Phase III	Student is seated, reclined against an incline of 30°. Student lifts head and teacher assists lifting of shoulders.
Phase IV	Student is seated, reclined against an incline of 30°. Student lifts head and shoulders.
Phase V	Student is seated, reclined against an incline of 10°. Student lifts head and teacher assists lifting of shoulders.
Phase VI	Student is seated, reclined against an incline of 10°. Student lifts head and shoulders.
Phase VII	Lying supine on floor, student lifts head and teacher assists lifting of shoulders.
Phase VIII	Lying supine on floor, student lifts head and shoulders up enough so teacher can slide hand under shoulder blades without resistance.
SUGGESTED MATERIALS:	Inclined surfaces 45°, 30°, and 10° from floor.
TEACHING NOTES:	1. Teaching Sequence — Teach this skill beginning with Phase I. Then teach Phases II through VIII. 2. *Caution:* This program requires modification by appropriate support personnel for use with students who have muscle tone problems, paralysis, or other physical handicaps.

Y. Pushes up on Extended Arms — Prone

Approximate Age for Skill Acquisition
6-7 months

TERMINAL OBJECTIVE: Lying prone, student will raise head and chest, pushing up on hands. Elbows remain straight.

PREREQUISITE SKILLS: When placed on extended arms, student must be able to bear weight for two seconds and to bear weight on elbows.

Phase I — Teacher gives student complete physical assistance at shoulders to raise head and chest. Teacher releases assistance fully and student rests full weight on hands. Elbows remain straight for two seconds.

Phase II — Teacher assists student to raise head and chest by lifting and releasing at student's shoulders. Student rests full weight on hands following each release. (Three lifts and releases for each trial.)

Phase III — Teacher assists student to raise head and chest by lifting or tapping gently under chin. Student pushes up and rests full weight on hands for two seconds.

Phase IV — Student raises head and chest, pushes up, and rests full weight on hands for two seconds.

SUGGESTED MATERIALS: A reinforcing toy or food.

TEACHING NOTES:
1. Teaching Sequence — Teach this skill beginning with Phase I. Then teach Phases II, III, and IV.
2. For Phase II, lifting and releasing should be conducted about four times for each trial.
3. In conducting each of the phases of this sequence, a reinforcing toy or food should be held near the top of the student's head.
4. *Caution:* This program requires modification by appropriate support personnel for use with students who have muscle tone problems, paralysis, or other physical handicaps.

Z. Protective Extension Forward on Ball or Bolster
Approximate Age for Skill Acquisition 6-7 months

TERMINAL OBJECTIVE:	When rolled to an upside down prone position on ball, student will extend arms, place open hands on floor and rest weight on hands.
PREREQUISITE SKILLS:	Student must be able to bear weight on extended arms, sitting and prone.
Phase I	Teacher #1 places student's hands on hers and holds student's elbows straight. Teacher #2 rolls student forward a few inches from floor, weight support partially on teacher #1's hands. Student does not withdraw hands when rolled forward.
Phase II	Teacher #1 places student's hands on hers and holds student's elbows straight. Teacher #2 rolls student forward a few inches from floor, weight support partially on Teacher #1's hands. Student pushes against Teacher #1's hands when rolled forward.
Phase III	Teacher #1 places student's hands on hers and holds student's elbows straight. Teacher #2 rolls student forward a few inches from floor, weight supported partially on Teacher #1's hands. Teacher #1 guides student's hands to floor, student does not withdraw hands when rolled forward.
Phase IV	Teacher #1 places student's hands on hers. Teacher #2 rolls student forward a few inches from floor, weight supported partially on Teacher #1's hands. Teacher #1 guides student's hands to floor, student pushes against floor when rolled forward.
Phase V	Teacher rolls student forward, student reaches for floor and rests weight on hands.
Phase VI	Teacher rolls student forward quickly, student extends hand and catches weight immediately.
SUGGESTED MATERIALS:	For large student, large inflated beach ball with

Gross Motor Skills

a 36- to 48-inch diameter; for small student, a 24- to 30-inch bolster or ball.

TEACHING NOTES:
1. Teaching Sequence — Teach this skill beginning with Phase I. Then teach Phases II through VI.
2. This sequence should be conducted by two teachers for Phases I through V.
3. Positioning for Phases I through IV: Student is placed in prone position on ball. Teacher #1 faces student. Teacher #2 holds student's legs from behind.
4. *Caution:* This program requires modification by appropriate support personnel for use with students who have muscle tone problems, paralysis, or other physical handicaps.

AA. Protective Extension — Forward

Approximate Age for Skill Acquisition
6-8 months

TERMINAL OBJECTIVE:	Student extends hands when body is moved quickly downward toward floor by teacher.
PREREQUISITE SKILLS:	Protective extension on ball; bears weight on extended arms; bears weight on elbows.
Phase I	Student extends arms when body is moved downward toward floor; teacher gives complete physical assistance for student to extend arms.
Phase II	Student extends arms when body is moved downward toward floor; teacher taps arms intermittently. Any attempt to extend arms is correct.
Phase III	Student extends arms when body is moved downward toward floor; teacher touches backs of arms simultaneously to initiate extension of arms.
Phase IV	Student extends arms when body is moved downward toward floor by teacher.
Phase V	Student extends arms when body is moved quickly downward toward floor by adult.
SUGGESTED MATERIALS:	None.
TEACHING NOTES:	1. Teaching Sequence — Teach this skill beginning with Phase I. Then teach Phase II, III, IV, and V.
2. Teacher should hold student horizontal to the floor and provide complete support to the student's body. Student's arms remain free.
3. *Caution:* This program requires modification by appropriate support personnel for use with students who have muscle tone problems, paralysis, or other physical handicaps.

BB. Rolls from Side Lying to Stomach

Approximate Age for Skill Acquisition
7-8 months

TERMINAL OBJECTIVE:	From side lying position, student reaches forward with top arm, brings head forward turning face down, and as roll is completed, lifts head and shoulder to free "down" arm.
PREREQUISITE SKILLS:	Head turns freely, lifts head in prone, bears weight on one elbow.
Phase I	Teacher gives complete physical assistance for student to move top shoulder forward (face turned down), lifts head and shoulder to free "down" arm.
Phase II	Teacher taps top shoulder forward (face turned down) and provides complete physical assistance to lift head and shoulder to free "down" arm.
Phase III	Teacher taps top shoulder forward to initiate roll and taps to initiate lifting of head and shoulder to free "down" arm. Student completes roll.
Phase IV	Teacher taps top shoulder forward to initiate roll. Student frees "down" arm and completes roll.
Phase V	From side lying position, student reaches forward with top arm, brings head forward turning face down, and as roll is completed, lifts head and shoulder to free "down" arm.
SUGGESTED MATERIALS:	Things that can be used as visual or auditory cues: bell, musical or noise toy, light, food, toys that are *both* visually and auditorily stimulating, voice of teacher.
TEACHING NOTES:	1. Teaching Sequence — Teach this skill beginning with Phase I. Then teach Phases II through V. 2. In teaching each of the phases, a visual or auditory object should be presented for the student to reach toward.

3. *Caution:* This program requires modification by appropriate support personnel for use with students who have muscle tone problems, paralysis, or other physical handicaps.

CC. Rolls from Back to Stomach

Approximate Age for Skill Acquisition
7-8 months

TERMINAL OBJECTIVE: From back lying position, student lifts head, turns face in direction of roll reaching across with "top" arm, turns head until face is down, lifts head and shoulder to free "down" arm and completes roll.

PREREQUISITE SKILLS: Rolls from side to stomach, lifts head supine, turns head freely, hands to midline supine, rolls from back to side.

Phase I: Teacher gives complete physical assistance for student to lift head, turn face in direction of roll reaching across with "top" arm, turn head until face is down, lift head and shoulder to free "down" arm and complete roll.

Phase II: Teacher taps student's forehead to lift head and turn face in direction of roll and for student to reach across with top arm, turn head until face is down, lift head and shoulder to free "down" arm and complete roll.

Phase III: Teacher taps student's forehead to lift head and turn face in direction of roll and taps student's shoulder to lift head and shoulder to free "down" arm and complete roll.

Phase IV: Teacher taps student's forehead to lift head and turn face in direction of roll and student independently lifts head and shoulder to free "down" arm and complete roll.

Phase V: From lying position, student lifts head, turns face in direction of roll reaching across with "top" arm, turns head until face is down, lifts head to free "down" arm and completes roll.

SUGGESTED MATERIALS: Things that can be used as visual or auditory cues: bells, musical or noise toy, light, food, toys that are *both* visually and auditorily stimulating, voice of teacher.

TEACHING NOTES: 1. Teaching Sequence — Teach this skill be-

ginning with Phase I. Then teach Phases II through V.
2. Within a given training session, student must work on rolling both to the right and to the left. Data should be maintained for both directions.
3. A visual or auditory object should be presented for student to reach forward to in all phases.
4. *Caution:* This program requires modification by appropriate support personnel for use with students who have muscle tone problems, paralysis, or other physical handicaps.

DD. Weight Bearing with Ball

Approximate Age for
Skill Acquisition
7-8 months

TERMINAL OBJECTIVE: Student bears weight on floor, touching ball with hands.

PREREQUISITE SKILLS: Props on elbows, lifts head prone, sits with support.

Phase I — Student is given weight-bearing stimulus by teacher pulling legs against her. Student bears weight against teacher for two seconds.

The following steps are to be used with Phase I:

Steps

1. Teacher in standing position. (Student bears weight on legs in horizontal position.)
2. Teacher in kneeling position. (Student bears weight on legs in 45° angle to floor).

Phase II — Student is rolled down so feet are touching floor, heels placed flat on floor by teacher. Support is given at student's knees while student rests weight on feet.

Phase III — Student is rolled down so feet are touching floor, heels placed flat on floor by teacher. Student lifts head off ball while he rests weight on feet and teacher supports at knees.

Phase IV — Student is rolled down so feet are touching floor, heels placed flat on floor by teacher. Student lifts head, neck, and chest off ball while he rests weight on feet and teacher supports at knees.

Phase V — Student is rolled down so feet are touching floor, heels placed flat on floor by teacher. Student raises upper torso off ball while he rests weight on feet and trainer supports at knees.

Phase VI — Student is rolled down so feet are touching floor, heels placed flat on floor by teacher. Upper torso is raised off ball and only thighs and hands are resting on ball as student rests

	weight on feet and teacher supports at knees.
Phase VII	Student is rolled down so feet are touching floor, heels placed flat on floor by teacher. Student is supported by touching hands on ball and trainer supports at knees.
Phase VIII	Student bears weight on floor. Teacher removes support from knees and assists balance from hips.
Phase IX	Student bears weight on floor touching ball with hands.

The following steps are to be used with Phases II through IX:

Steps

1. Time of 2 seconds.
2. Time of 4 seconds.
3. Time of 6 seconds.
4. Time of 8 seconds.
5. Time of 10 seconds.
6. Time of 15 seconds.
7. Time of 20 seconds.
8. Time of 25 seconds.
9. Time of 30 seconds.
10. Time of 40 seconds.
11. Time of 50 seconds.
12. Time of 60 seconds.
13. Time of 90 seconds.
14. Time of 120 seconds (2 minutes).

SUGGESTED MATERIALS: Large inflated beachball with a 36- to 48-inch diameter. For a very small child, a 24-inch ball may be easier.

TEACHING NOTES:
1. Teaching Sequence — Teach this skill beginning with Phase I, Step 1. Then teach Phase I, Step 2 before teaching Phase II, Steps 1 through 14 and Phase III, Steps 1 through 14. Continue to teach remaining phases and steps in the same manner.
2. A second teacher may be needed for safety to prevent sideways falls and to keep ball from rolling away from student.
3. Positioning for Phases II through VII — Student is placed in prone position on ball with legs extended and feet placed on either side of teacher's body. Student's knees are rotated out by teacher, and support is given at the student's knees. Time is measured

from beginning of placement in required position until student collapses or withdraws.
4. *Caution:* This program requires modification by appropriate support personnel for use with students who have muscle tone problems, paralysis, or other physical handicaps.

EE. Sits without Support

Approximate Age for
Skill Acquisition
7-8 months

TERMINAL OBJECTIVE:	Student sits on flat surface without support for five minutes.
PREREQUISITE SKILLS:	Sits with support, independent head control.
Phase I	Student sits on flat surface, teacher holding lower hips.
Phase II	Student sits on flat surface, teacher holding thighs parallel to floor.
Phase III	Student sits on flat surface without support.

The following steps are to be used with Phases I, II, and III:

Steps

1. 5 seconds.
2. 10 seconds.
3. 15 seconds.
4. 20 seconds.
5. 30 seconds.
6. 40 seconds.
7. 50 seconds.
8. 60 seconds.
9. 90 seconds.
10. 120 seconds.
11. 180 seconds.
12. 240 seconds.
13. 300 seconds.

SUGGESTED MATERIALS: Student's favorite toys or visually stimulating toys for student to look at (necessary if steps 6 through 13 are used).

TEACHING NOTES:

1. Teaching Sequence — Teach this skill beginning with Phase I, Step 1. Then teach Phase I, Steps 2 through 5 before teaching Phase II, Steps 1 through 5. Continue to teach the remaining phases and steps in the same manner. Steps 6 through 13 should only be used if student is engaged in activity (looking at or playing with toys for specified time period) but should definitely be part of Phase III.
2. *Caution:* This program requires modification by appropriate support personnel for use with students who have muscle tone problems, paralysis, or other physical handicaps.

FF. Stands with Support

Approximate Age for
Skill Acquisition
7-9 months

TERMINAL OBJECTIVE: When placed standing, student will support own weight and maintain balance with abdomen and hands in contact with waist level support for three minutes.

PREREQUISITE SKILLS: Bears weight on elbows and extended arms; sits with support; weight bearing with ball.

Phase I — Teacher assists student to maintain hands on support and keep hips, knees, and back straight.

Phase II — Teacher assists to keep hips, knees, and back straight, student maintains hands on support.

Phase III — Teacher assists to keep hips and back straight, student maintains hands on support.

Phase IV — Teacher assists to keep hips straight, student maintains hands on support.

Phase V — Student maintains hands on support and stands without assistance.

Phase VI — Student recovers position on support when teacher taps abdomen 2 to 3 inches away from support. Teacher does not hold student but catches if necessary.

The following steps are to be used with Phases I through VI:

<u>Steps</u>

1. Maintains position for 2 seconds.
2. Maintains position for 3 seconds.
3. Maintains position for 4 seconds.
4. Maintains position for 5 seconds.
5. Maintains position for 7 seconds.
6. Maintains position for 10 seconds.
7. Maintains position for 15 seconds.
8. Maintains position for 20 seconds.
9. Maintains position for 30 seconds.
10. Maintains position for 45 seconds.
11. Maintains position for 60 seconds.

12. Maintains position for 90 seconds.
13. Maintains position for 120 seconds.
14. Maintains position for 150 seconds.
15. Maintains position for 180 seconds.

SUGGESTED MATERIALS: Table, foot stool, or other stable support of waist height.

TEACHING NOTES:
1. Teaching Sequence — Teach this skill beginning with Phase I, Steps 1 through 15. Then teach Phases II, Steps 1 through 15 and continue with all remaining phases in the same manner.
2. *Caution:* This program requires modification by appropriate support personnel for use with students who have muscle tone problems, paralysis, or other physical handicaps.

GG. Pivots on Stomach

Approximate Age for
Skill Acquisition
7-9 months

TERMINAL OBJECTIVE:	Student pivots on stomach, moving body in left or right arc for 180°.
PREREQUISITE SKILLS:	Bears weight on elbows, shifts weight on elbows.
Phase I	Student lifts upper trunk. While supported on arms/hands, he moves body to left, pushing against floor with arms/hands when given complete physical assistance by teacher. Repeat to right side. Move arms in direction of movement of pivot once each.
Phase II	Student lifts upper trunk. While supported on arms/hands, he moves body to left, pushing against floor with arms/hands when teacher pushes against student's shoulders in appropriate direction and moves hands alternately. Repeat to right side.
Phase III	Student lifts upper trunk. While supported on arms/hands, he moves body to left, pushing against floor with arms/hands when teacher taps student's shoulders in appropriate direction. Repeat to right side.
Phase IV	Student lifts upper trunk. While supported on arms/hands, he moves body to left, pushing against floor with arms/hands. Repeat to right side.

The following steps apply to Phases II through IV:

Steps

1. Moves arms in direction of movement of pivot two times each.
2. One-fourth arc (90°).
3. One-half arc (180°).

SUGGESTED MATERIALS:	Toys to which student can move.
TEACHING NOTES:	1. Teaching Sequence — Teach this skill beginning with Phase I. Then teach Phase II,

Steps 1 through 3 before teaching Phase III, Steps 1 through 3. Continue to teach remaining phase and steps in the same manner.
2. Positioning for Phases I through IV — student is in prone position.
3. Teacher moves reinforcer in direction of pivot just out of reach of student.
4. *Caution:* This program requires modification by appropriate support personnel for use with students who have muscle tone problems, paralysis, or other physical handicaps.

HH. Lifts Abdomen in Prone Position Approximate Age for
Skill Acquisition
8-9 months

Terminal Objective: Student pushes up on extended arms. Then student lifts abdomen with no object behind feet. Student's knees may remain on floor or lift off. Maintains position for ten seconds.

Prerequisite Skills: Bears weight on extended arms, sits with support, has head control.

Phase I   Student pushes up on extended arms. Then student lifts abdomen and pushes with feet against a solid object with teacher providing complete physical assistance.

Phase II   Student pushes up on extended arms. Then student lifts abdomen and pushes with feet against a solid object with teacher lifting student's abdomen and releasing, but holding feet against solid object.

Phase III   Student pushes up on extended arms. Then student lifts abdomen and pushes with feet against a solid object with teacher holding feet against solid object.

Phase IV   Student pushes up on extended arms. Then student lifts abdomen, pushing with feet against a solid object.

Phase V   Student pushes up on extended arms. Then student lifts abdomen with no object behind feet. Student's knees may remain on floor or lift off.

The following steps are to be used with Phases I through V:

Steps

1. One second.
2. Two seconds.
3. Three seconds.
4. Four seconds.
5. Five seconds.
6. Ten seconds.

SUGGESTED MATERIALS: A wall can be used as the solid object.

TEACHING NOTES:
1. Teaching Sequence — Teach this skill beginning with Phase I, Step 1. Then teach Phase I, Steps 2 through 6 before teaching Phase II, Steps 1 through 6. Continue to teach remaining phases and steps in same manner.
2. *Caution:* This program requires modification by appropriate support personnel for use with students who have muscle tone problems, paralysis, or other physical handicaps.

II. Bears Weight on Hands and Knees When Placed

Approximate Age for Skill Acquisition
8-9 months

TERMINAL OBJECTIVE: When placed on hands and knees, student will remain in position and bear weight on hands and knees for sixty seconds.

PREREQUISITE SKILLS: Bears weight on extended arms, has head control.

Phase I — Teacher places student on hands and knees, providing complete physical assistance for student to bear weight and support head.

Phase II — Teacher places student on hands and knees and provides complete physical assistance for student to bear weight. Student supports head.

Phase III — Teacher places student on hands and knees and provides support at hips. Student maintains weight and balance on hands.

Phase IV — Teacher places student on hands and knees and provides support at knees. Student maintains weight and balance on hands. Teacher taps as necessary to assist student in maintaining balance.

Phase V — Teacher places student on hands and knees and provides support at knees. Student maintains weight and balance on hands.

Phase VI — When placed on hands and knees, student will remain in position and bear weight on hands and knees.

The following steps are to be used with Phases I through VI:

Steps
1. Five seconds.
2. Ten seconds.
3. Fifteen seconds.
4. Twenty seconds.
5. Thirty seconds.
6. Forty seconds.
7. Fifty seconds.
8. Sixty seconds.

SUGGESTED MATERIALS: Visual or auditory toys or attractions to keep student's attention.

TEACHING NOTES:
1. Teaching Sequence — Teach this skill beginning with Phase I, Step 1. Then teach Phase I, Steps 2 through 8 before teaching Phase II, Steps 1 through 8. Continue to teach remaining phases and steps in the same manner.
2. *Caution:* This program requires modification by appropriate support personnel for use with students who have muscle tone problems, paralysis, or other physical handicaps.

JJ. Bears Weight on One Extended Arm and Reaches — Hands and Knees

Approximate Age for Skill Acquisition
8-10 months

TERMINAL OBJECTIVE:	From four-point kneeling (hands and knees), student reaches forward with one hand to touch or take object while sustaining weight of upper trunk on extended arm.
PREREQUISITE SKILLS:	Bears weight on one arm and reaches. Bears weight on hands and knees. Reaches for objects.
Phase I	From hands and knees, student reaches forward with one hand, bearing weight on other extended arm. Teacher assists weight shift at shoulders and stabilizes at shoulders and hips as student reaches. Repeat procedure with opposite arm.
Phase II	From hands and knees, student reaches forward with one hand, bearing weight on other on extended arm. Teacher assists weight shift at shoulder and stabilizes at hips and waist as student reaches. Repeat procedure with opposite arm.
Phase III	From hands and knees, student reaches forward with one hand, bearing weight on other extended arm. Teacher assists weight shift at shoulder and stabilizes at hips as student reaches. Repeat procedure with opposite arm.
Phase IV	From hands and knees, student reaches forward with one hand, bearing weight on other extended arm. Teacher stabilizes at hips as student reaches. Repeat procedure with opposite arm.
Phase V	From hands and knees, student reaches forward with one hand, bearing weight on other extended arm. Student reaches without assistance. Repeat procedure with opposite arm.
SUGGESTED MATERIALS:	Toys for which student can reach.

TEACHING NOTES:
1. Teaching Sequence — Teach Phase I. Then teach Phases II through V.
2. Purpose of this program is to develop weight shift for creeping.
3. A phase is successful if student is able to reach for toy and either touch or retrieve it without losing balance.
4. *Caution:* This program requires modification by appropriate support personnel for use with students who have muscle tone problems, paralysis, or other physical handicaps.

KK. Moves toward an Object

Approximate Age for
Skill Acquisition
9-10 months

TERMINAL OBJECTIVE: Student moves toward an object presented at a 5-foot distance within his field of vision, responding within ten seconds.

PREREQUISITE SKILLS: Student must have some type of movement. See Teaching Note #2.

Phase I Student moves toward an object placed 3 inches beyond his reach when given complete physical assistance.

Phase II Student moves toward an object placed 3 inches beyond his reach given a physical prompt from the teacher to initiate movement. Student responds within thirty seconds.

Phase III Student moves toward an object placed 3 inches beyond his reach, responds within thirty seconds.

Phase IV Student moves toward an object placed 3 inches beyond his reach, responds within twenty seconds.

Phase V Student moves toward an object, responds within ten seconds.

The following steps are to be used with Phase V only:

<u>Steps</u>

1. Object presented 3-inch distance beyond student's reach.
2. Object presented 6-inch distance beyond student's reach.
3. Object presented 9-inch distance beyond student's reach.
4. Object presented 12-inch distance beyond student's reach.
5. Object presented 2-foot distance beyond student's reach.
6. Object presented 3-foot distance beyond student's reach.
7. Object presented 4-foot distance beyond student's reach.
8. Object presented 5-foot distance beyond student's reach.

SUGGESTED MATERIALS: Toy or object that is pleasing to student.

TEACHING NOTES: 1. Teaching Sequence — Teach this skill beginning with Phase I. Then teach Phases II

through IV before teaching Phase V, Steps 1 through 8.
2. The type of movement the student exhibits is entirely dependent upon the skill level of the student. Teacher should specify acceptable response from each particular student, i.e. movement of arms, crawling, etc.
3. The object of this program is to have the student first move toward an object at a 3-inch distance and then increase the distance that he moves.
4. *Caution:* This program requires modification by appropriate support personnel for use with students who have muscle tone problems, paralysis, or other physical handicaps.

LL. Moves Forward Down Ramp

Approximate Age for
Skill Acquisition
9-10 months

TERMINAL OBJECTIVE: Beginning from a prone position (head down on ramp), student uses any pattern of movement (except rolling) to move forward down ramp.

PREREQUISITE SKILLS: Bears weight on elbows, weight shift on forearms, sitting with support.

Phase I Foot end of ramp is raised high enough that smallest movement will start student down ramp. Student uses any pattern of movement to move forward down ramp.

Phase II Foot end of ramp is raised to 75 percent of the height in Phase I. Student uses any pattern of movement to move forward down ramp.

Phase III Foot end of ramp is raised to 50 percent of the height in Phase I. Student uses any pattern of movement to move forward down ramp.

Phase IV Foot end of ramp is raised to 25 percent of the height in Phase I. Student uses any pattern of movement to move forward down ramp.

Phase V Foot end of ramp is raised to 10 percent of the height in Phase I. Student uses any pattern of movement to move forward down ramp.

The following steps are to be used with Phases I through V:

<u>Steps</u>

1. Student placed 1 foot from bottom of ramp.
2. Student placed 2 feet from bottom of ramp.
3. Student placed 3 feet from bottom of ramp.
4. Student placed 4 feet from bottom of ramp.
5. Student placed 5 feet from bottom of ramp.
6. Student placed 6 feet from bottom of ramp.

SUGGESTED MATERIALS: Sheet of ¾-inch plywood for ramp, covered with material or vinyl. Toys to which the student can move.

TEACHING NOTES:
1. Teaching Sequence — Teach this skill beginning with Phase I, Step 1. Then teach Phase I, Steps 2 through 6 before teaching Phase II, steps 1 through 6. Continue to teach remaining phases and steps in the same manner.
2. Positioning for Phases I through V — Student is placed prone, head down, on ramp.
3. Teacher should position herself at the bottom of the ramp to catch student should he fall. A second teacher may be needed to prevent a fall from the sides of the ramp.
4. *Caution:* This program requires modification by appropriate support personnel for use with students who have muscle tone problems, paralysis, or other physical handicaps.

MM. Crawls Forward on Floor　　　Approximate Age for
　　　　　　　　　　　　　　　　　　　Skill Acquisition
　　　　　　　　　　　　　　　　　　　9-10 months

TERMINAL OBJECTIVE:	Student crawls 5 feet forward on stomach moving legs, hips, trunk, and arms.
PREREQUISITE SKILLS:	Bears weight on one elbow and reaches, sits with support, moves forward down ramp, pivots on stomach.
Phase I	Given complete physical assistance to move, student crawls forward on stomach moving hands/arms and legs.
Phase II	Given physical assistance to move hips, legs, and trunk, student crawls forward on stomach moving arms.
Phase III	Given physical assistance to move hips and legs, student crawls forward on stomach moving trunk and arms.
Phase IV	Given physical assistance to move legs, student crawls forward on stomach moving hips, trunk, and arms.
Phase V	When teacher pushes against student's feet, student crawls forward on stomach moving legs, hips, trunk, and arms.
Phase VI	Student crawls forward on stomach moving legs, hips, trunk, and arms.

The following steps apply to Phases I through VI:

Steps

1. 3 inches.
2. 6 inches.
3. 9 inches.
4. 12 inches.
5. 15 inches.
6. 18 inches.
7. 2 feet.
8. 3 feet.
9. 4 feet.
10. 5 feet.

SUGGESTED MATERIALS:	Reinforcing toy or people to which the student can move.
TEACHING NOTES:	1. Teaching Sequence — Teach this skill beginning with Phase I, Step 1. Then teach

Phase I, Steps 2 through 10 before teaching Phase II, Steps 1 through 10. Teach remaining phases and steps in the same manner.

2. *Caution:* This program requires modification by appropriate support personnel for use with students who have muscle tone problems, paralysis, or other physical handicaps.

NN. Leans and Regains Balance, Sitting Position

Approximate Age for Skill Acquisition
9-10 months

TERMINAL OBJECTIVE:	Student leans over 6 inches in any direction (forward, backward, left, or right), regains balance, and returns to original upright sitting position.
PREREQUISITE SKILLS:	Supported sitting.
Phase I	Student leans over while sitting and, with complete physical assistance around entire trunk, returns to upright position.
Phase II	Student leans over while sitting and, with physical assistance to return halfway to upright position, returns remainder of way.
Phase III	Student leans over while sitting and, with physical assistance to return one-fourth of the way to upright position, returns remainder of way.
Phase IV	Student leans over in specified direction (forward, backward, left, or right), regains balance, and returns to original upright sitting position.

The following steps apply to all of the phases:

Steps

1. Leans forward 6 inches.
2. Leans to right side 6 inches.
3. Leans to left side 6 inches.
4. Leans backward 6 inches.

SUGGESTED MATERIALS:	Favorite toy or food to which the student can lean. (Teacher may have to assist student to pick up or grasp object, but this gives purpose for this movement and makes it more functional for student.)
TEACHING NOTES:	1. Teaching Sequence — Teach this skill beginning with Phase I, Step 1. Then teach Phase I, Steps 2 through 4 before teaching Phase II, Steps 1 through 4. Continue to

teach remaining phases and steps in the same manner.
2. Student does not have to be sitting independently to begin this program. It should be initiated as soon as head control and supported sitting are in student's repertoire. The purpose of this program is not to teach independent sitting, but rather to build and strengthen trunk righting reactions and/or equilibrium reactions while in a sitting position.
3. Cue should involve two verbal directions: (a) "Get the toy," "Move it," "Lean forward," "Lean backward," or "Lean to the side." Teacher may provide additional touch to indicate direction student should lean. (b) "Sit back up."
4. Distances as prescribed in the steps may be modified to relate to size of student.
5. Generalization procedures should begin as soon as student reaches Phase III by placing him in a free operant setting and presenting stimuli to initiate these behaviors, such as toys or food.
6. *Caution:* This program requires modification by appropriate support personnel for use with students who have muscle tone problems, paralysis, or other physical handicaps.

OO. Protective Extension — Lateral

Approximate Age for
Skill Acquisition
9-10 months

TERMINAL OBJECTIVE: Student will extend hand and arm to each side when pushed sideways from sitting position.

PREREQUISITE SKILLS: Bears weight on extended arms, sits with support.

Phase I With student in sitting position on floor or wide bench, student is tipped to side from shoulder at approximately 45° angle. Teacher assists with placement of hand and holds elbow straight so student holds weight. Repeat for other side.

Phase II With student in sitting position on floor or wide bench, student is tipped to side from shoulder at approximately 45° angle. Teacher assists with placement of hand. Student holds elbow straight. Repeat for other side.

Phase III With student in sitting position on floor or wide bench, student is tipped to side from shoulder at approximately 45° angle. Teacher assists by tapping arm out until it is extended. Repeat for other side.

Phase IV Teacher tips student from shoulder. Student catches self. Repeat for other side.

SUGGESTED MATERIALS: If a wide bench is used, its length should be approximately three times student's hip width.

TEACHING NOTES:
1. Teaching Sequence — Teach this skill beginning with Phase I, then teach Phase II before teaching Phases III and IV.
2. This sequence should be taught for both sides of body. Data should be maintained for each side.
3. As student catches self with one hand and arm, the opposite arm and leg may fly up. This is normal. *Do not restrict this movement.*
4. *Caution:* This program requires modification by appropriate support personnel for

use with students who have muscle tone problems, paralysis, or other physical handicaps.

PP. Gets to Sitting from Prone Approximate Age for
Skill Acquisition
9-10 months

TERMINAL OBJECTIVE: Student gets to sitting position from prone by pushing abdomen up with hands and/or arms, bending legs and knees, placing weight on left or right side of hips, and pushing trunk upright into sitting position.

PREREQUISITE SKILLS: Sits without support, bears weight on extended arms, maintains hands and knees, lifts abdomen in prone position, leans and regains balance.

Phase I Teacher gives complete physical assistance to student to get to sitting position from prone by pushing abdomen up with hands and/or arms, bending legs and knees, placing weight on left or right side of hips, and pushing trunk upright into sitting position.

Phase II Teacher gives physical assistance to student to get to sitting position from prone by pushing abdomen up with hands and/or arms, bending legs and knees, and placing weight on left or right side of hips. Teacher begins upward movement of student's trunk; student completes movement and sits upright.

Phase III Teacher gives physical assistance to student to get to sitting position from prone by pushing abdomen up with hands and/or arms, bending legs and knees and placing weight on left or right side of hips. Student pushes trunk upright into sitting position independently.

Phase IV Teacher gives physical assistance to student to get to sitting position from prone by pushing abdomen up with hands and/or arms and bending legs and knees. Student places weight on left or right side of hips and pushes trunk upright into sitting position independently.

Phase V Teacher gives physical assistance to student to get to sitting position from prone by pushing

	abdomen up with hands and/or arms. Student bends legs and knees, places weight on left or right side of hips, and pushes trunk upright into sitting position independently.
Phase VI	Student gets to sitting position from prone, pushing abdomen up with hands and/or arms. Student bends legs and knees, places weight on left or right side of hips, and pushes trunk upright into sitting position.
SUGGESTED MATERIALS:	May use attention-getting toy or food to direct movement.
TEACHING NOTES:	1. Teaching Sequence — Teach this skill beginning with Phase I. Then teach Phase II through VI. 2. *Caution:* This program requires modification by appropriate support personnel for use with students who have muscle tone problems, paralysis, or other physical handicaps.

QQ. Gets to Hands and Knees

Approximate Age for
Skill Acquisition
9-10 months

TERMINAL OBJECTIVE:	Student will get to hands and knees from prone position by raising abdomen, pulling knees under, and pushing up to extended arms given physical cue (tap under abdomen). Student holds position for five seconds.
PREREQUISITE SKILLS:	Student can maintain a four-point kneel when placed for at least five seconds, bears weight on extended arms, sits without support.
Phase I	From prone position, teacher lifts hips, pulls student back onto knees, and with hand under chest, assists student to push up on arms. Student maintains for five seconds.
Phase II	From prone position, teacher lifts hips and pulls student back onto knees. Once knees are placed, student pushes up on arms. Student maintains for five seconds.
Phase III	From prone position, teacher lifts hips slightly, student pulls knees under and lifts up on arms. Student maintains for five seconds.
Phase IV	With physical cue (tap under abdomen), student raises abdomen, pulls knees under, and pushes up to extended arms. Student maintains for five seconds.
SUGGESTED MATERIALS:	None.
TEACHING NOTES:	1. Teaching Sequence — Teach this skill beginning with Phase I. Then teach Phases II through IV. 2. *Caution:* This program requires modification by appropriate support personnel for use with students who have muscle tone problems, paralysis, or other physical handicaps.

RR. Gets to Sitting from Hands and Knees

Approximate Age for Skill Acquisition 9-10 months

TERMINAL OBJECTIVE:	From kneeling position, student sits back on heels, puts weight on left or right side of hips, places weight on buttocks, and straightens legs to assume sitting position.
PREREQUISITE SKILLS:	Sits without support, maintains hands and knees.
Phase I	From kneeling position, student is given complete physical assistance from teacher to sit back on heels, to put weight on left or right side of hips, to place weight on buttocks, and to straighten legs.
Phase II	From kneeling position, student is given complete physical assistance by teacher to sit back on heels, to put weight on left or right side of hips, to place weight on buttocks. Student straightens legs independently.
Phase III	From kneeling position, student is given complete physical assistance by teacher to sit back on heels and to put weight on left or right side of hips. Student places weight on buttocks and straightens legs independently.
Phase IV	From kneeling position, student is given complete physical assistance by teacher to sit back on heels. Student puts weight on left or right side of hips, places weight on buttocks, and straightens legs independently.
Phase V	From kneeling position, student sits back on heels, puts weight on left or right side of hips, places weight on buttocks, and straightens legs to assume sitting position.
SUGGESTED MATERIALS:	None.
TEACHING NOTES:	1. Teaching Sequence — Teach this skill beginning with Phase I. Then teach Phases II through V.

2. Teach sitting to both right and left within each training session. Record separate data for left and right sides.
3. *Caution:* This program requires modification by appropriate support personnel for use with students who have muscle tone problems, paralysis, or other physical handicaps.

SS. Pulls to Kneel Stand

Approximate Age for Skill Acquisition
9-11 months

TERMINAL OBJECTIVE: Student pulls from sitting position to kneel stand position, hands placed on a support and hips raised into full extension. Student holds position for five seconds.

PREREQUISITE SKILLS: Sits without support, bears weight on extended arms.

Phase I — Teacher gives full assistance to place student's hands on support, to bend legs to side sitting position, and to lift hips into full extension. Student holds kneel stand position.

Phase II — Student places hands on support. Teacher bends legs to side-sitting position and lifts hips into full extension. Student holds kneel stand position.

Phase III — Student places hands on support. Teacher bends legs to side sitting position and lifts slightly under shoulders. Student raises hips into full extension and holds kneel stand position.

Phase IV — Student places hands on support. Teacher taps legs to bend into side sitting position. Student pulls to kneel stand and holds position independently.

Phase V — Student pulls from sitting position to kneel stand position, hands placed on a support and hips raised into full extension. Student holds position.

The following steps are to be used with Phases I through V:

Steps

1. Two seconds.
2. Three seconds.
3. Four seconds.
4. Five seconds.

SUGGESTED MATERIALS: Stable support that is waist to chest high to student when he is kneeling in an upright position. If a plywood support is used, it can be covered with a soft vinyl fabric to ensure a smooth and comfortable surface for teaching this skill.

TEACHING NOTES:

1. Teaching Sequence — Teach this skill beginning with Phase I, Step 1. Then teach Phase I, Steps 2 through 4 before teaching Phase II, Steps 1 through 4. Teach all subsequent phases and steps in the same manner.
2. The student begins by sitting on the floor with legs extended out in front of him.
3. *Caution:* This program requires modification by appropriate support personnel for use with students who have muscle tone problems, paralysis, or other physical handicaps.

TT. Independent Weight Bearing — Grasp

Approximate Age for Skill Acquisition 9-12 months

TERMINAL OBJECTIVE: Student bears weight without grasping objects for 2 minutes.

PREREQUISITE SKILLS: Sit without support, kneel at support, weight bear on arms, stands with support.

Phase I — Student bears weight and grasps solid object with two hands.

The following steps are to be used with Phase I:

Steps

1. 2 seconds.
2. 4 seconds.
3. 6 seconds.
4. 8 seconds.
5. 10 seconds.
6. 15 seconds.
7. 20 seconds.
8. 25 seconds.
9. 30 seconds.
10. 40 seconds.
11. 50 seconds.
12. 60 seconds.
13. 90 seconds.
14. 120 seconds.
15. 150 seconds.

Phase II — Ten months. Student bears weight and grasps flexible hose with two hands.

The following steps are to be used with Phase II:

Steps

1. 5 seconds.
2. 10 seconds.
3. 15 seconds.
4. 20 seconds.
5. 30 seconds.
6. 40 seconds
7. 50 seconds.
8. 60 seconds.
9. 90 seconds.
10. 120 seconds.
11. 150 seconds.
12. 180 seconds.

Phase III — Student bears weight and grasps flexible hose with either right or left hand 3 inches from the teacher's hand.

Phase IV — Eleven months. Student bears weight and grasps flexible hose with either right or left hand 6 inches from teacher's hand.

Phase V — Student bears weight and grasps flexible hose

	with either right or left hand 9 inches from teacher's hand.
Phase VI	Student bears weight and grasps flexible hose with either right or left hand 12 inches from teacher's hand.
Phase VII	Student bears weight and grasps flexible hose with either right or left hand 18 inches from teacher's hand.
Phase VIII	Twelve months. Student bears weight and grasps flexible hose with either right or left hand twenty-four inches from teacher's hand.
Phase IX	Student bears weight and grasps flexible hose with either right or left hand 30 inches from teacher's hand.
Phase X	Student bears weight and grasps flexible hose with either right or left hand 36 inches from teacher's hand.

The following steps are to be used with Phases IV through X:

Steps

1. 15 seconds.
2. 20 seconds.
3. 30 seconds.
4. 40 seconds.
5. 50 seconds.
6. 60 seconds.
7. 90 seconds.
8. 120 seconds.
9. 150 seconds.
10. 180 seconds.

Phase XI	Student bears weight without grasping objects.

The following steps are to be used with Phase XI:

Steps

1. 3 seconds.
2. 6 seconds.
3. 9 seconds.
4. 12 seconds.
5. 15 seconds.
6. 20 seconds.
7. 25 seconds.
8. 30 seconds.
9. 40 seconds.
10. 50 seconds.
11. 60 seconds.
12. 80 seconds.
13. 100 seconds.
14. 120 seconds.

SUGGESTED MATERIALS:	Solid object (Phase II), such as wall-mounted bar, chair with adult sitting in it, length of flexible garden hose about 40 inches long.
TEACHING NOTES:	1. Teaching Sequence — Teach this skill beginning with Phase I, Step 1. Then teach Phase I, Steps 2 through 15 before teaching Phase II, Steps 1 through 12. Continue to teach the remaining phases and steps in the same manner.
2. This program should be taught for students who have a grasping ability. If the student is unable to grasp, use program UU.
3. Student may or may not need mechanical support braces.
4. In order for a student to maintain a weight-bearing position for more than ten seconds, reinforcers should probably be delivered either continuously or at a frequent intermittent schedule while student is maintaining weight-bearing position.
5. *Caution:* This program requires modification by appropriate support personnel for use with students who have muscle tone problems, paralysis, or other physical handicaps.

UU. Standing — No Grasp Ability

Approximate Age for Skill Acquisition
9-12 months

TERMINAL OBJECTIVE: Child stands without support for 2 minutes when positioned by teacher.

PREREQUISITE SKILLS: Sits without support, head control, weight bearing with ball.

Phase I — Nine months. Teacher supports student from behind in standing position supporting knees, hips, and trunk at chest level.

Phase II — Nine months. Teacher supports student from behind in standing position supporting knees, hips, and trunk from waist level.

Phase III — Nine months. Teacher supports student from behind in standing position supporting knees and hips.

Phase IV — Nine months. Teacher supports student from behind in standing position with hands around thighs to keep knees straight.

Phase V — Ten months. Teacher holds hands near student's hips to balance. Student supports own weight.

Phase VI — Ten months. Teacher holds both student's hands for balance, student supports own weight.

Phase VII — Eleven months. Teacher holds one hand for balance, student supports own weight.

Phase VIII — Twelve months. Student stands without support when positioned by teacher.

The following steps are to be used with Phases I through VIII:

Steps

1. Stands for 2 seconds.
2. Stands for 3 seconds.
3. Stands for 4 seconds.
4. Stands for 5 seconds.
5. Stands for 7 seconds.
6. Stands for 10 seconds.
7. Stands for 15 seconds.
8. Stands for 20 seconds.
9. Stands for 30 seconds.
10. Stands for 45 seconds.

11. Stands for 60 seconds.
12. Stands for 90 seconds.
13. Stands for 120 seconds.

SUGGESTED MATERIALS: None.

TEACHING NOTES:
1. Teaching Sequence — Teach this skill beginning with Phase I, Steps 1 through 13. Then teach Phase II, Steps 1 through 13 before teaching Phase III, Steps 1 through 13. Continue to teach remaining phases in the same manner.
2. If student has grasping ability, use program TT. This program is for students who are unable to grasp.
3. Note age norms for phases.
4. Positioning for Phases — Teacher supports student with knees or feet bracing student's feet, one hand at student's knees. Teacher's body supports hips and other hand supports trunk.
5. *Caution:* This program requires modification by appropriate support personnel for use with students who have muscle tone problems, paralysis, or other physical handicaps.

VV. Lifts Trunk with Hands and Arms   Approximate Age for
Skill Acquisition
9-12 months

TERMINAL OBJECTIVE: Student lifts trunk with hands and arms when supported by ankles, prone position. Maintains position for ten seconds.

PREREQUISITE SKILL: Skill II, "Attains and maintains weight bearing on elbow, prone."

Phase I Student lifts trunk while in a prone position, pushing with hands and arms; teacher provides physical assistance to raise trunk to 45° angle and maintains support on student's hands.

Phase II Student lifts trunk while in prone position, pushing with hands and arms; teacher provides physical assistance to raise trunk to 45° angle, student maintains support on own hands.

Phase III Student lifts trunk while in prone position pushing with hands and arms, teacher supports student at hips.

Phase IV Student lifts trunk while in prone position, pushing with hands and arms; teacher supports child by thighs.

Phase V Student lifts trunk while in prone position, pushing with hands and arms; adult supports student by knees.

Phase VI Student lifts trunk while in prone position, pushing with hands and arms, teacher supports student by ankles.

The following steps are to be used with Phases III through VI:

Steps

1. Maintains position for one second.
2. Maintains position for two seconds.
3. Maintains position for three seconds.
4. Maintains position for four seconds.
5. Maintains position for five seconds.

6. Maintains position for seven seconds.
7. Maintains position for ten seconds.

SUGGESTED MATERIALS: None.

TEACHING NOTES:
1. Teaching Sequence — Teach this skill beginning with Phase I. Then teach Phase II before teaching Phase III, Steps 1 through 7. Then teach Phase IV, Steps 1 through 7 and continue to teach remaining phases and steps in the same manner.
2. *Caution:* This program requires modification by appropriate support personnel for use with students who have muscle tone problems, paralysis or other physical handicaps.

WW. Creeps on Hands and Knees   Approximate Age for
                                              Skill Acquisition
                                               10-12 months

TERMINAL OBJECTIVE: Student creeps forward on a flat, level surface 5 feet to desired object.

PREREQUISITE SKILLS: Ability to maintain balance on hands and knees, can shift weight on extended arms, sits without support.

Phase I   Student creeps forward six inches on hands and knees with complete assistance from teacher to move hands and knees.

Phase II   Student creeps forward 6 inches on hands and knees with teacher moving hand and pulling behind shoulder to encourage knees to move.

Phase III   Student creeps forward on hands and knees. Teacher moves knee well forward and pushes forward gently, student moves hands.

Phase IV   Student creeps forward, teacher tapping forward gently to initiate creeping movement.

Phase V   Student creeps forward on a flat, level surface independently.

The following steps are to be used with Phases III through V:

<u>Steps</u>

1. 6 inches.
2. 1 foot.
3. 2 feet.
4. 3 feet.
5. 4 feet.
6. 5 feet.

SUGGESTED MATERIALS: None.

TEACHING NOTES: 1. Teaching Sequence — Teach this skill beginning with Phase I. Then teach Phase II. Then teach Phase III, Steps 1 through 6 before teaching Phase IV, Steps 1 through 6. Continue to teach the remaining phases and steps in the same manner.

2. Cross pattern creep (reciprocal — one hand then opposite leg moves) is *not* required for correct response, but is preferable. However, specific pattern must be established for student so that consistent programming can be conducted.
3. *Caution:* This sequence requires modification by appropriate support personnel for use with students who have muscle tone problems, paralysis, or other physical handicaps.

XX. Turns Trunk in Sitting Position

Approximate Age for Skill Acquisition 10-12 months

TERMINAL OBJECTIVE:	While sitting, student will turn shoulders enough to reach across the midline to take object presented 6 inches to one side of the opposite shoulder.
PREREQUISITE SKILLS:	Ability to sit independently, protective extension laterally; leans and regains balance; hands cross midline
Phase I	While sitting, student waves and moves arms independently. May bat at a balloon suspended in front of him. Do with both hands and with each hand singly.
Phase II	While sitting, student reaches forward to object with one hand. Teacher may gently restrain other hand or give student a toy to hold to occupy that hand so student will reach with a specific hand.
Phase III	While sitting, student reaches across midline to object halfway from midline to lateral line with one hand. Teacher may gently restrain other hand or give student a toy to hold to occupy that hand so student will reach with a specific hand.
Phase IV	While sitting, student will turn shoulders enough to reach across the midline to take object presented 6 inches to one side of the opposite shoulder.
SUGGESTED MATERIALS:	Toys, suspended balloon.
TEACHING NOTES:	1. Teaching Sequence — Teach this skill beginning with Phase I. Then teach Phases II through IV. 2. This program must be run with both right hand and left hand within a single program session. Record separate data for left and right hands.

3. Student may support with hand not reaching.
4. Reinforcing object should be placed at arm's length from student.
5. The position of the objects for the various phases is as follows:
   a. Position for Phases I and II is to have the student face in the direction of arrow and reach for the object at A.

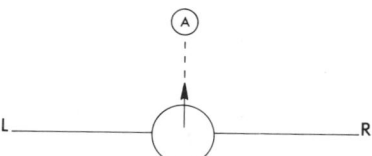

   b. Position for Phase III is to have the student face in the direction of arrow and reach for object A with the right hand and object B with the left hand.

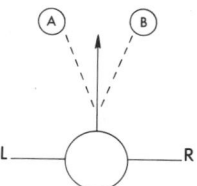

   c. Position for Phase IV is to have the student face in the direction of the arrow and reach for object A with the right hand and object B with the left hand.

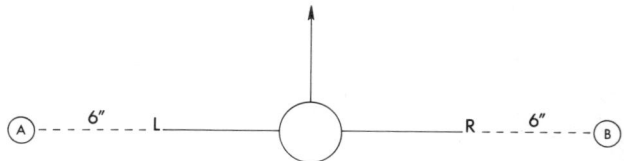

6. *Caution:* This program requires modification by appropriate support personnel for use with students who have muscle tone problems, paralysis, or other physical handicaps.

Gross Motor Skills 145

YY. Gets to Standing from Hands and Knees   Approximate Age for
Skill Acquisition
10-16 months

TERMINAL OBJECTIVE: From hands and knees, student places hands on floor, places feet in weight-bearing position, and rises to standing position unassisted.

PREREQUISITE SKILLS: Stands with support, sits without support in supported kneel standing, bears weight on hands and knees, shifts weight.

Phase I   From hands and knees, student raises one hand and places it on platform of designated height.

Phase II   From hands and knees, student raises one hand and places it on platform of designated height. Teacher provides assistance to help maintain hand while student raises other hand and places it on platform.

Phase III   From hands and knees, student raises one hand to platform of designated height and maintains it there without help while placing other hand on platform.

The following steps are to be used with Phases I through III:

Steps

1. Platform is 1 inch high.
2. Platform is 2 inches high.
3. Platform is 3 inches high.
4. Platform is 4 inches high.
5. Platform is 5 inches high.
6. Platform is 6 inches high.
7. Platform is 7 inches high.
8. Platform is 8 inches high.
9. Platform is 9 inches high.
10. Platform is 10 inches high.
11. Platform is 11 inches high.
12. Platform is 12 inches high.

Phase IV   From hands and knees, student raises both hands to platform of designated height. Teacher assists student to standing.

Phase V   From hands and knees, student raises both hands to platform of designated height, flexes one hip, and places that foot in weight-bearing position. Teacher assists student to complete standing.

Phase VI	From hands and knees, student raises both hands to platform of designated height, flexes one hip, and places that foot in weight-bearing position. Student pushes up until second foot is placed so weight is supported on both feet. Teacher assists student to complete standing.
Phase VII	From hands and knees, student places hands on platform of designated height, places feet in weight-bearing position. With teacher assistance at shoulders and hips, student rises to standing position.
Phase VIII	From hands and knees, student places hands on platform of designated height, places feet in weight-bearing position. With teacher assisting from hips only, student rises to standing position.
Phase IX	From hands and knees, student places hands on platform of designated height and places feet in weight-bearing position. With teacher with hand on back assisting for balance only, student rises to standing position.
Phase X	From hands and knees, student places hands on platform of designated height, places feet in weight-bearing position, and rises to standing position, teacher only touching him on back.
Phase XI	From hands and knees, student places hands on platform of designated height, places feet in weight-bearing position and rises to standing position unassisted.

The following steps are to be used with Phases IV through IX:

Steps

1. Platform is 20 inches high.
2. Platform is 18 inches high.
3. Platform is 16 inches high.
4. Platform is 14 inches high.
5. Platform is 12 inches high.
6. Platform is 10 inches high.
7. Platform is 8 inches high.
8. Platform is 6 inches high.
9. Platform is 4 inches high.
10. Platform is 2 inches high.
11. Platform is 1 inch high.
12. Hand on floor is 0 inches high.

SUGGESTED MATERIALS: Platform with adjustable height.

TEACHING NOTES:
1. Teach this skill beginning with Phase I, Steps 1 through 12. Then teach Phase II, Steps 1 through 12 before teaching Phase III, Steps 1 through 12. Continue to teach the remaining phases and steps in the same manner.
2. *Caution:* This program requires modification by appropriate support personnel for use with students who have muscle tone problems, paralysis, or other physical handicaps.

ZZ. Gets to Sitting from Supine

Approximate Age for Skill Acquisition 11-12 months

TERMINAL OBJECTIVE: Student gets into a sitting position from supine.

PREREQUISITE SKILLS: Sits independently, rolls to side from supine, bears weight on extended arms.

Note: Student cannot do sit-up without hands generally until age six. Sit-ups with legs straight are hazardous for back.

Phase I — Student rolls to side from supine position. Teacher completely assists student to sitting with one or both hands by holding hips on floor and pulling student around and up with shoulder.

Phase II — Student rolls to side from supine position. Teacher assists student to sit with one or both hands by holding hips on floor and pulling child around with shoulder. Student pushes up to sitting.

Phase III — Student rolls to side from supine position. Teacher assists student with one or both hands, holding hips on floor. Student pulls trunk over and pushes up to sitting.

Phase IV — Student rolls to side from supine position. Teacher assists student by tapping in appropriate direction with one or both hands. Student pushes up to sitting.

Phase V — Student gets into sitting position from supine independently.

SUGGESTED MATERIALS: None.

TEACHING NOTES:
1. Teaching Sequence — Teach this skill beginning with Phase I. Then teach Phase II before teaching Phases III through V.
2. *Caution:* This program requires modification by appropriate support personnel for use with students who have muscle tone problems, paralysis, or other physical handicaps.

AAA. Creeps on Hands and Knees, Negotiating Environment

Approximate Age for Skill Acquisition
10-14 months

TERMINAL OBJECTIVE: Student creeps on hands and knees up and down stairs, over obstacles, up and down an inclined surface, in and out of large containers, and through a tunnel.

PREREQUISITE SKILLS: Ability to creep on flat surface.

Phase I — Student creeps on hands and knees given complete physical assistance.

Phase II — Student creeps on hands and knees given physical assistance three-fourths of the way through task. Student completes last one-fourth alone.

Phase III — Student creeps on hands and knees given physical assistance halfway through task. Student completes last half alone.

Phase IV — Student creeps on hands and knees given physical assistance one-fourth of the way through task. Student completes last three-fourths alone.

Phase V — Student creeps on hands and knees.

The following steps are to be used with Phases I through V:

Steps

1. Down an inclined surface.
2. Up an inclined surface.
3. Through a tunnel/barrel.
4. Over an obstacle (adult's legs, blocks, small inner tube, etc.).
5. Out of a container (cardboard box, laundry basket, etc.).
6. Into container.

SUGGESTED MATERIALS: Inclined surface made of sturdy plastic or plywood. Surface should be covered with fabric protector. Large toy tunnel, large cardboard box, large laundry basket.

TEACHING NOTES: 1. Teaching Sequence — Teach this skill beginning with Phase I, Step 1. Then teach

Phases II through V, Step 1 before teaching Phases I through V, Step 2. Continue to teach each step with all phases before going on to the next step.
2. After all steps have been learned, they may be combined in a number of ways to become a type of obstacle course.
3. *Caution:* This program requires modification by appropriate support personnel for use with students who have muscle tone problems, paralysis or other physical handicaps.

BBB. Cruises Approximate Age for
Skill Acquisition
10-14 months

TERMINAL OBJECTIVE:	Student cruises ten side steps along an object using hands, arms, and/or any part of body as support.
PREREQUISITE SKILLS:	Ability to stand when positioned by trainer at object.
Phase I	Student cruises along solid, large object using any part of body as support. Teacher gives complete physical assistance to student to shift weight and move leading foot and following foot. Repeat to opposite side.
Phase II	Student cruises along large object using any part of body as support. Teacher gives physical assistance to student to shift weight and move leading foot. Student moves following foot. Repeat to opposite side.
Phase III	Student cruises along solid, large object using any part of body as support. Teacher gives physical assistance to student to shift weight. Student moves leading and following foot. Repeat to opposite side.
Phase IV	Student cruises along solid, large object using any part of body as support. Teacher gives tap to leading foot so student sidesteps. Repeat to opposite side.
Phase V	Student cruises along solid, large object using any part of body as support. Teacher touches student's shoulders to initiate movement. Repeat to opposite side.
Phase VI	Student cruises along large, solid object. Repeat to opposite side.
Phase VII	Student cruises along a low level opened object. Repeat to opposite side.
Phase VIII	Student cruises along a wall. Repeat to opposite side.

The following steps apply to all of the phases:

Steps

1. One side step.
2. Two side steps.
3. Three side steps.
4. Four side steps.
5. Five side steps.
6. Six side steps.
7. Seven side steps.
8. Eight side steps.
9. Nine side steps.
10. Ten side steps.

SUGGESTED MATERIALS: Phases I through VI. Solid large object includes items such as a sofa; large, weighted cardboard box; storage chest; trunk; etc. that are waist to chest high.

Phase VII. A low level opened object is one providing less stability and support for the student's body. Items such as a coffee table, child-height classroom table, bed, bookshelves, etc. Objects used should be found in the child's environment, either classroom or home, that are waist to chest high.

Phase VIII. Wall.

TEACHING NOTES:
1. Teaching Sequence — Teach this skill beginning with Phase I, Step 1. Then teach Phase I, Steps 1 through 10, followed by Phase II, Steps 1 through 10. Continue teaching remaining phases and steps in a similar order.
2. Cruising is movement on feet, usually sideways, using a solid object for support.
3. Teach cruising to both right and left each training session. Record separate data for left and right sides.
4. In order to achieve a side step the student must shift his weight twice. For instance, if he is side-stepping to the right, he must first shift his body weight to the left to pick up his right foot, then shift his weight back to the right after he has advanced his right foot in order for him to follow with his left foot.
5. *Caution:* This program requires modification by appropriate support personnel for use with students who have muscle tone problems, paralysis, or other physical handicaps.

CCC. Independent Movement — Grasp   Approximate Age for
Skill Acquisition
11-16 months

TERMINAL OBJECTIVE: Student moves forward without physical support, 25 feet.

PREREQUISITE SKILLS: Weight bearing with support, weight shift in standing.

Phase I   Eleven months. Student moves forward, bearing his own weight and requires solid object and both hands for support.

Phase II   Eleven months. Student moves forward, bearing his own weight and requires flexible support and both hands. Hands of child on hose are spaced at distance equal to width of shoulders. Teacher's hands are 3 inches from outside of student's hands on hose.

Phase III   Twelve months. Student moves forward, bearing own weight and requires flexible support (hose) with either right or left hand. Hose is held by teacher at a distance of 3 inches from student's hands.

Phase IV   Student moves forward, bearing own weight and requires flexible support (hose) with either right or left hand. Hose is held by teacher at a distance of 6 inches from student's hands.

Phase V   Student moves forward, bearing own weight and requires flexible support (hose) with either right or left hand. Hose is held by teacher at a distance of 9 inches from student's hands.

Phase VI   Student moves forward, bearing own weight, requires flexible support (hose) with either right or left hand. Hose is held by teacher at a distance of 12 inches from student's hands.

Phase VII   Student moves forward, bearing his own weight, holding with one hand a flexible hose approximately 8 inches long.

Phase VIII   Twelve months. Student moves forward without physical support.

The following steps apply to Phases I through VIII:

Steps

1. Distance of 1 foot.
2. Distance of 2 feet.
3. Distance of 3 feet.
4. Distance of 4 feet.
5. Distance of 6 feet.
6. Distance of 8 feet.
7. Distance of 10 feet.
8. Distance of 13 feet.
9. Distance of 16 feet.
10. Distance of 20 feet.
11. Distance of 25 feet.

SUGGESTED MATERIALS: Solid object chest high for Phase I, such as a chair or a broomstick held by teacher. Flexible hose for Phases II through VIII. Flexible hose should be approximately 1 inch in diameter (one 15 inches long, one 8 inches long).

TEACHING NOTES:
1. Teaching Sequence — Teach this skill beginning with Phase I, Steps 1 through 11 before teaching Phase II, Steps 1 through 11. Continue to teach the remaining phases and steps in the same manner.
2. When using flexible hose, be sure that student is not leaning forward so that teacher is "holding him up." The student should be bearing his own weight and using the hose to help him sustain his balance. To facilitate this the teacher should let the student pace his advancement rather than pulling him forward.
3. In Phases III through VI, the dominant hand of the student should be holding the hose. The teacher holds the hose with the same hand.
4. This program is designed for students who have the ability to grasp. For students who cannot grasp or who have difficulty grasping, use program DDD.
5. *Caution:* This program requires modification by appropriate support personnel for use with students who have muscle tone problems, paralysis, or other physical handicaps.

DDD. Walking — No Grasp Ability

Approximate Age for Skill Acquisition
11-16 months

TERMINAL OBJECTIVE:	Student walks forward without physical support, 25 feet.
PREREQUISITE SKILLS:	Bears full weight, sits without support.
Phase I	Eleven months. Student walks forward with teacher supporting him under the arms. Student takes full weight on feet.
Phase II	Student walks forward with teacher supporting both hands (teacher holds on top of student's wrists).
Phase III	Student walks forward with teacher holding one hand.
Phase IV	Student walks forward with teacher holding front of shirt.
Phase V	Twelve months. Student walks forward without support.

The following steps apply to Phases I through V:

Steps
1. Distance of 1 foot.
2. Distance of 2 feet.
3. Distance of 3 feet.
4. Distance of 4 feet.
5. Distance of 6 feet.
6. Distance of 8 feet.
7. Distance of 10 feet.
8. Distance of 13 feet.
9. Distance of 16 feet.
10. Distance of 20 feet.
11. Distance of 25 feet.

SUGGESTED MATERIALS: None.

TEACHING NOTES:
1. Teaching Sequence — Teach this skill beginning with Phase I, Step 1. Then teach Phase I, Steps 2 through 11 before teaching Phase II, Steps 1 through 11. Continue to teach remaining phases in the same manner.
2. This program is designed for the student who cannot grasp or who has great diffi-

culty grasping. For the student who is able to grasp, use program CCC.
3. *Caution:* This program requires modification by appropriate support personnel for use with students who have muscle tone problems, paralysis, or other physical handicaps.

EEE. Gets to Sitting from Standing Appropriate Age for Skill Acquisition 12-13 months

TERMINAL OBJECTIVE:	Student sits from standing without support.
PREREQUISITE SKILLS:	Stands with support, moves legs separately.
Phase I	Student places hands on waist-high support and sits on floor with full assistance from teacher to maintain hands, to balance from shoulder, to support trunk, to kneel to one knee, and to guide hips to sit back to side of supporting knee.
Phase II	Student maintains hands on waist-high support. Teacher balances from shoulder, supports trunk, assists kneeling to one knee, guiding hips to sit back to side of supporting knee.
Phase III	Student maintains hands on waist-high support. Teacher balances from shoulder, assists kneeling to one knee, and guides hips to sit back to side of supporting knee.
Phase IV	Student maintains hands on waist-high support. Teacher assists kneeling to one knee and guides hips to sit back to side of supporting knee.
Phase V	Student maintains hands on waist-high support. Teacher assists kneeling to one knee. Student completes sitting.
Phase VI	Student maintains hands and sits after kneeling on one knee. Teacher taps leg and hip to cue toward direction student is to sit.
Phase VII	Student sits with tap on leg from teacher.
Phase VIII	Student sits with support surface lowered to 75 percent of height in Phase I.
Phase IX	Student sits with support surface lowered to 50 percent of height in Phase I.
Phase X	Student sits with support surface lowered to 25 percent of height in Phase I.

Phase XI	Student sits with support surface lowered to 10 percent of height in Phase I.
Phase XII	Student puts hands on floor and sits from standing without assistance.
SUGGESTED MATERIALS:	Solid support — table, sofa, chair, or adjustable platform. Cushions may be used.

TEACHING NOTES:	1. Teaching Sequence — Teach Phase I before teaching Phase II and then teach all succeeding phases.
	2. A student under two years of age may drop backward directly to sitting. This is acceptable. For safety, do the program on an exercise mat.
	3. Alternate sequence:
	  Phase I Student drops to sitting with teacher assisting to keep head forward and to bend hips and knees.
	  Phase II Student drops to sitting with teacher tapping shoulder and hips.
	  Phase III Student drops to sitting with teacher touching shoulder only.
	  Phase IV Student sits from standing without assistance.
	4. *Caution:* This program requires modification by appropriate support personnel for use with students who have muscle tone problems, paralysis, or other physical handicaps.

FFF. Sits in Chair

Approximate Age for
Skill Acquisition
12-16 months

TERMINAL OBJECTIVE: When placed in appropriate sized chair, student will sit without using hands for support for sixty seconds. Feet remain on floor.

PREREQUISITE SKILLS: Sits without support.

Phase I — When placed in chair, student sits with teacher supporting student at hips and shoulders. Feet remain on floor.

Phase II — When placed in chair, student sits with teacher supporting student at hips. Feet remain on floor.

Phase III — When placed in chair, student will sit without using hands for support. Feet remain on floor.

The following steps are to be used with Phases I through III:

Steps
1. Five seconds.
2. Ten seconds.
3. Fifteen seconds.
4. Twenty seconds.
5. Twenty-five seconds.
6. Thirty seconds.
7. Forty seconds.
8. Fifty seconds.
9. Sixty seconds.

SUGGESTED MATERIALS: Appropriate-sized chair for all phases and small toy for student to play with during program.

TEACHING NOTES:
1. Teaching Sequence — Teach this skill beginning with Phase I, Step 1. Then teach Phase I, Steps 2 through 9 before teaching Phase II, Steps 1 through 9. Continue to teach remaining phases and steps in the same manner.
2. Give small toy to occupy hands during program.
3. *Caution:* This program requires modification by appropriate support personnel for use with students who have muscle tone problems, paralysis, or other physical handicaps.

GGG. Gets Up from a Chair

Approximate Age for Skill Acquisition
12-16 months

TERMINAL OBJECTIVE:	Student gets up from a chair and stands.
PREREQUISITE SKILLS:	Independent weight bearing, pushes up on extended arms.
Phase I	When seated in a chair, student scoots buttocks forward to edge of seat; using arms to push, student lifts trunk up and stands, given complete physical assistance by teacher.
Phase II	When seated in a chair, student scoots buttocks forward to edge of seat; using arms to push, student lifts trunk up given physical assistance by teacher. Student stands without assistance.
Phase III	When seated in a chair, student scoots buttocks forward to edge of seat given physical assistance by teacher. Student lifts trunk up and stands without assistance.
Phase IV	When seated in a chair, student gets up from a chair and stands.
SUGGESTED MATERIALS:	Chair, short enough so student's feet at least touch floor.
TEACHING NOTES:	1. Teaching Sequence — Teach this skill beginning with Phase I. Then teach Phases II through IV. 2. *Caution:* This program requires modification by appropriate support personnel for use with students who have muscle tone problems, paralysis, or other physical handicaps.

HHH. Falls Forward Approximate Age for
Skill Acquisition
13-16 months

TERMINAL OBJECTIVE: Student falls forward from a kneel stand position, catching weight of body on arms.

PREREQUISITE SKILLS: Props on extended arms, protective extension on ball.

Phase I When pushed gently on back by teacher, student falls forward from a kneel stand position, catching self with both arms/hands and given complete physical assistance by teacher to support student's arms and under chest.

Phase II When pushed gently on back by teacher, student falls forward from a kneel stand position. Teacher pushes arms of student out in front, student catches weight of body.

Phase III When pushed gently on back by teacher, student falls forward from a kneel stand position, catching weight of body on extended arms.

SUGGESTED MATERIALS: None.

TEACHING NOTES:
1. Teaching Sequence — Teach this skill beginning with Phase I. Then teach Phases II and III.
2. *Caution:* This program requires modification by appropriate support personnel for use with students who have muscle tone problems, paralysis, or other physical handicaps.

III. Gets into a Chair

Approximate Age for
Skill Acquisition
13-20 months

TERMINAL OBJECTIVE: Student gets into appropriate-sized chair, seated facing forward, with legs out in front.

PREREQUISITE SKILLS: Standing independently.

Phase I Standing in front of chair with back facing chair, student places back of thighs against seat of the chair and pushes body back into chair, using arms to assist. Complete physical assistance given by teacher.

Phase II Student places back of thighs against seat of the chair and pushes body halfway back into the chair, given complete physical assistance by teacher. Student completes motion into the back of the chair.

Phase III Student places back of thighs against seat of the chair and starts body onto chair, given complete physical assistance by teacher. Student pushes back into seat of chair.

Phase IV Student places back of thighs against the seat of the chair, given physical assistance by teacher; student sits on chair.

Phase V Student gets into chair, seated facing forward, with legs out in front.

SUGGESTED MATERIALS: Appropriate-sized chair that is short enough so student's feet can touch floor.

TEACHING NOTES:
1. Teaching Sequence — Teach this skill beginning with Phase I, then teach Phases II through V.
2. Student should be reaching behind him to locate chair. This reaching behind will normally require him to bend his knees and lean forward. This movement should be included when given complete assistance.
3. *Caution:* This program requires modification by appropriate support personnel for use with students who have muscle tone problems, paralysis, or other physical handicaps.

JJJ. Walks Up Incline

Approximate Age for
Skill Acquisition
14-17 months

TERMINAL OBJECTIVE: Student moves forward 8 feet, bearing his own weight up an inclined surface placed four stairs high off floor.

PREREQUISITE SKILLS: Walks forward without support.

Phase I — Student moves forward, bearing his own weight up an inclined surface placed one stair high off floor.

Phase II — Student moves forward, bearing his own weight up an inclined surface placed two stairs high off floor.

Phase III — Student moves forward, bearing his own weight up an inclined surface placed three stairs high off floor.

Phase IV — Student moves forward, bearing his own weight up an inclined surface placed four stairs high off floor.

The following steps are to be used with Phases I through IV:

Steps

1. Distance of 2 feet.
2. Distance of 3 feet.
3. Distance of 4 feet.
4. Distance of 6 feet.
5. Distance of 8 feet.

SUGGESTED MATERIALS: 1-inch plywood, 8 feet long, cut to a width so that one end of plywood can be rested on floor and other end on stairs. A flight of stairs four or more high.

TEACHING NOTES:
1. Teaching Sequence — Teach this skill beginning with Phase I, Step 1. Then teach Phase I, Steps 2 through 5 before teaching Phase II, Steps 1 through 5. Continue to teach remaining phases and steps in the same manner.
2. Incline must not be slippery.

3. *Caution:* This program requires modification by appropriate support personnel for use with students who have muscle tone problems, paralysis, or other physical handicaps.

KKK. Kneels

Approximate Age for
Skill Acquisition
14-18 months

TERMINAL OBJECTIVE: Student bears weight on both knees, keeping trunk in an upright position and legs bent at the knees in a 90° angle and maintains position for ten seconds.

PREREQUISITE SKILLS: Extension of arms and ability to lift trunk with hands and arms.

Phase I Student bears weight on both knees, keeping trunk in an upright position and legs bent at the knees in a 90° angle. Teacher provides complete physical assistance.

Phase II Student bears weight on both knees, keeping trunk in an upright position and legs bent at the knees in a 90° angle. Teacher provides physical assistance to keep student's trunk upright. Student keeps legs at 90° angle.

Phase III Student bears weight on both knees, keeping trunk in an upright position and legs bent at the knees in a 90° angle. Teacher provides support to keep trunk upright by holding student's arms.

Phase IV Student bears weight on both knees keeping trunk in an upright position and legs bent at the knees in a 90° angle. Teacher provides support to keep trunk upright by holding one of student's arms.

Phase V Student bears weight on both knees keeping trunk in an upright position and legs bent at the knees in a 90° angle.

The following steps are to be used with Phases I through V:

Steps
1. Maintains position for one second.
2. Maintains position for two seconds.
3. Maintains position for three seconds.
4. Maintains position for four seconds.
5. Maintains position for five seconds.

6. Maintains position for seven seconds.
7. Maintains position for ten seconds.

SUGGESTED MATERIALS: None.

TEACHING NOTES:
1. Teaching Sequence — Teach this skill beginning with Phase I, Step 1. Then teach Phase I, Steps 2 through 7, before teaching Phase II, Steps 1 through 7. Continue to teach all steps with one phase before going on to next phase.
2. *Caution:* This program requires modification by appropriate support personnel for use with students who have muscle tone problems, paralysis, or other physical handicaps.

LLL. Bears Weight on One Knee — Half-Kneeling Position

Approximate Age for Skill Acquisition 14-18 months

TERMINAL OBJECTIVE: Student bears weight on one knee while in a half-kneeling position for ten seconds.

PREREQUISITE SKILLS: Student is capable of kneeling.

Phase I Student remains in half-kneeling position, one leg with knee on floor, the other leg bent at the knee in a 90° angle with foot flat on floor. Complete physical assistance given by teacher to maintain position. Repeat to opposite side.

Phase II Student remains in half-kneeling position, one leg with knee on floor, the other leg bent at the knee in a 90° angle with foot flat on floor. Teacher holds both student's hands. Repeat to opposite side.

Phase III Student remains in half-kneeling position, one leg with knee on floor, the other leg bent at the knee in a 90° angle with foot flat on floor. Teacher holds one of student's hands. Repeat to opposite side.

Phase IV Student remains in half-kneeling position, one leg with knee on floor, the other leg bent at the knee in a 90° angle with foot flat on floor. Physical assistance given to initiate position. Teacher leaves hands touching both student's legs while student maintains position. Repeat to opposite side.

Phase V Student remains in half-kneeling position, one leg with knee on floor, the other leg bent at the knee in a 90° angle with foot flat on floor, physical assistance given to initiate position. Teacher touches upper leg to maintain position. Repeat to opposite side.

Phase VI Student remains in half-kneeling position, one leg with knee on floor, the other leg bent at the knee in a 90° angle with foot flat on floor, physical assistance given to initiate position. Student maintains alone. Repeat to opposite side.

Phase VII   Student bears weight on one foot while in a half kneeling position. Repeat to opposite side.

The following steps are to be used with Phases I through V:

Steps

1. One second.
2. Two seconds.
3. Three seconds.
4. Four seconds.
5. Five seconds.
6. Seven seconds.
7. Ten seconds.

SUGGESTED MATERIALS: Padded rug or gym mat to kneel on.

TEACHING NOTES:

1. Teaching Sequence — Teach this skill beginning with Phase I, Step 1. Then teach Phase I, Steps 2 through 7 before teaching Phase II, Steps 1 through 7. Continue to teach all steps with one phase before going on to the next phase.

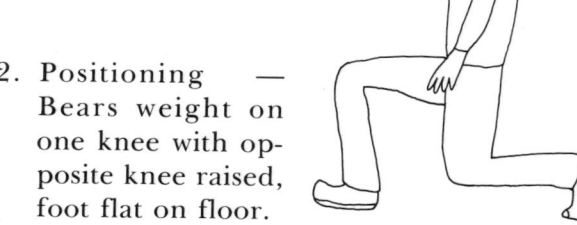

2. Positioning — Bears weight on one knee with opposite knee raised, foot flat on floor.
3. Left and right knee should be done during each teaching session, with separate data recorded for each knee.
4. *Caution:* This program requires modification by appropriate support personnel for use with students who have muscle tone problems, paralysis, or other physical handicaps.

MMM. Creeps up Steps

Approximate Age for
Skill Acquisition
15-17 months

TERMINAL OBJECTIVE: Child creeps up flight of four stairs.

PREREQUISITE SKILLS: Ability to creep independently, pull to stand.

Phase I — Place student with knees on one step and hands on next higher. Teacher raises one knee to same step as hand and lifts same hand forward to next higher step. Repeat same procedure for opposite knee and hand.

Phase II — Place student with knees on one step and hands on next higher. Teacher raises one knee to same step as hand, and student moves hand with teacher tapping for cue to next higher step. Repeat same procedure for opposite knee and hand.

Phase III — Place student with knees on one step and hands on next higher. Teacher raises one knee to same step as hand, and student lifts hand independently to next step. Repeat same procedure for opposite knee and hand.

Phase IV — Place student with knees on one step and hands on next higher. Teacher taps knee and student moves to next higher step. (Either hand going up to next step is acceptable.) Repeat tapping procedure to initiate movement for opposite knee.

Phase V — Place student with knees on one step and hands on next higher. Student moves hands and knees with verbal cue only. Any pattern of movement is acceptable.

The following steps apply to Phases I through V:

Steps
1. One stair.
2. Two stairs.
3. Three stairs.
4. Four stairs.

SUGGESTED MATERIALS: Small stair (3-inch rise) is preferable. Other stairs can be used if smaller stair is not available.

TEACHING NOTES:
1. Updating — Teach this skill beginning with Phase I, Step 1. Then teach Phase I, Steps 2 through 4, before teaching Phases II, Steps 1 through 4. Teach all subsequent phases and steps in the same manner.
2. Teacher may add more stairs to program, depending on how many steps are required in home or school setting.
3. *Caution:* This program requires modification by appropriate support personnel for use with students who have muscle tone problems, paralysis, or other physical handicaps.

NNN. Rides on Ride-On Toy Approximate Age for
Skill Acquisition
15-20 months

TERMINAL OBJECTIVE:	Student rides ride-on toy forward and backward 10 feet.
PREREQUISITE SKILLS:	Ability to grasp handles; ability to move feet back and forth.
Phase I	Student rides backward, holding on to handles. Teacher provides complete physical assistance.
Phase II	Student rides backward holding on to handles. Teacher provides physical assistance to start backward motion of toy. Student continues alone.
Phase III	Student rides backward on ride-on toy.
Phase IV	Student rides forward, teacher providing complete physical assistance to hold hands on handles and push with feet.
Phase V	Student rides forward, teacher providing complete physical assistance to hold hands on handles and start forward motion of toy. Student continues alone.
Phase VI	Student rides forward, teacher providing complete physical assistance to hold hands on handles. Student moves ride-on toy forward.
Phase VII	Student rides forward on ride-on toy.

The following steps are to be used with Phases I through VII:

Steps
1. 1 foot.
2. 2 feet.
3. 3 feet.
4. 4 feet.
5. 5 feet.
6. 10 feet.

SUGGESTED MATERIALS:	Ride-on toys that require pushing with feet. Pedals or moveable steering handles are not necessary. (Little Tykes® brand.)

TEACHING NOTES:
1. Teaching Sequence — Teach this skill beginning with Phase I, Step 1. Then teach Phase I, Steps 2 through 6 before teaching Phase II, Steps 1 through 6. Continue to teach all steps with one phase before going on to next phase.
2. Any method of foot movement is acceptable (moving feet together or alternately) providing student goes in correct direction. For consistency, teacher can identify which movement is most successful for student and specify it on the program so volunteer knows exactly how to assist student.
3. *Caution:* This program requires modification by appropriate support personnel for use with students who have muscle tone problems, paralysis, or other physical handicaps.

OOO. Walks Backward

Approximate Age for
Skill Acquisition
16-18 months

TERMINAL OBJECTIVE:	Student walks backward for five steps independently.
PREREQUISITE SKILLS:	Walks independently.
Phase I	Student walks backward with teacher holding arm of student and tapping legs alternately.
Phase II	Student walks backward with teacher holding arms of student for support.
Phase III	Student walks backward with teacher touching arms of child lightly.
Phase IV	Student walks backward independently.

The following steps apply to Phase 1 through IV:

Steps

1. One step.
2. Two steps.
3. Three steps.
4. Four steps.
5. Five steps.

SUGGESTED MATERIALS: None.

TEACHING NOTES:
1. Teaching Sequence — Teach this skill beginning with Phase I, Step 1. Then teach Phase I, Steps 2 through 5 before teaching Phase II, Steps 1 through 5. Teach all subsequent phases and steps in the same manner.
2. *Caution:* This program requires modification by appropriate support personnel for use with students who have muscle tone problems, paralysis, or other physical handicaps.

PPP. Walks Down Incline

Approximate Age for Skill Acquisition
16-18 months

TERMINAL OBJECTIVE: Student moves forward 8 feet, bearing his own weight down an inclined surface placed four stairs off floor.

PREREQUISITE SKILLS: Independent walking.

Phase I — Student moves forward bearing own weight down an inclined surface placed one stair high off floor.

Phase II — Student moves forward bearing own weight down an inclined surface placed two stairs high off floor.

Phase III — Student moves forward bearing own weight on inclined surface placed three stairs high off floor.

Phase IV — Student moves forward bearing own weight on inclined surface placed four stairs high off floor.

The following steps are to be used with Phases I through IV:

Steps
1. Distance of 2 feet.
2. Distance of 3 feet.
3. Distance of 4 feet.
4. Distance of 6 feet.
5. Distance of 8 feet.

SUGGESTED MATERIALS: 1-inch plywood, 8 feet long, cut to a width so that one end of plywood can be rested on floor and other end on stairs. A flight of stairs. Incline must not be slippery.

TEACHING NOTES:
1. Teaching Sequence — Teach this skill beginning with Phase I, Step 1. Then teach Phase I, Steps 2 through 5 before teaching Phase II, Steps 1 through 5. Continue to teach remaining phases and steps in the same manner.

2. *Caution:* This program requires modification by appropriate support personnel for use with students who have muscle tone problems, paralysis, or other physical handicaps.

QQQ. Creeps Down Stairs

Approximate Age for Skill Acquisition
18-20 months

TERMINAL OBJECTIVE:	Student gets on hands and knees at top of stairs and creeps down five steps backward without assistance.
PREREQUISITE SKILLS:	Creeps up stairs. Gets to hands and knees.
Phase I	When placed at top of stairs, student gets on hands and knees and creeps down stairs backward with complete physical assistance from teacher.
Phase II	Teacher assists student to turn and brings student's knees down. Student moves hands.
Phase III	Teacher assists student to turn and taps knees to come down. Student moves hands.
Phase IV	Teacher assists student to turn, student creeps down, with teacher tapping hands and knees to prevent turning and to control speed of descent.
Phase V	Teacher taps shoulder to initiate turn. Student creeps down steps without assistance.
Phase VI	Student gets on hands and knees at top of stairs and creeps down stairs backward without assistance.

The following steps apply to each of the phases:

Steps

1. One step.
2. Two steps.
3. Three steps.
4. Four steps.
5. Five steps.

SUGGESTED MATERIALS:	Flight of five to six steps, standard rise.
TEACHING NOTES:	1. Teaching Sequence — Teach this skill beginning with Phase I, Step 1; then teach Phase I, Steps 2 through 5 before teaching Phase II, Steps 1 through 5. Then teach

Phases III through VI in the same manner.
2. Teacher may adjust number of steps to correspond with situation in school or home.
3. *Caution:* This program requires modification by appropriate support personnel for use with students who have muscle tone problems, paralysis, or other physical handicaps.

RRR. Walks Up Stairs

Approximate Age for Skill Acquisition
18-36 months

TERMINAL OBJECTIVE:	Student walks up six steps, alternating feet, without the handrail or the aid of the teacher's hand.
PREREQUISITE SKILLS:	Walks independently, creeps up stairs.
Phase I	Eighteen months. Student walks up stairs holding on to handrail with one hand and teacher's hand with the other hand, utilizing a walking-type rhythm wherein he moves one foot up the stairs and moves the other foot even with that foot before proceeding to the next step. If he chooses to alternate feet, do not restrict.
Phase II	Twenty-four months. Student walks up steps holding on to handrail without aid of a teacher's hand and utilizing a walking-type rhythm wherein he moves one foot up the stairs and moves the other foot even with that foot before proceeding to the next step. If he chooses to alternate feet, do not restrict.
Phase III	Twenty-five months. Student walks up steps without holding on to handrail and without aid of teacher's hand, utilizing a walking type rhythm wherein he moves one foot up the stairs and moves the other foot even with that foot before proceeding to the next step. If he chooses to alternate feet, do not restrict.
Phase IV	Thirty months. Student walks up steps by holding on to handrail with one hand and teacher's hand with the other hand, alternating steps.
Phase V	Thirty-three months. Student walks up steps by holding on to handrail without aid of teacher's hand and alternating steps.
Phase VI	Thirty-six months. Student walks up steps, alternating feet, without the handrail or aid of adult's hand.

The following steps are to be used with Phases I through VI:

Steps

1. Two steps.
2. Three steps.
3. Four steps.
4. Five steps.
5. Six steps.

SUGGESTED MATERIALS: Flight of six stairs, standard rise stairs.

TEACHING NOTES:
1. Teaching Sequence — Teach this skill beginning with Phase I, Step 1. Then teach Phase I, Steps 2 through 5 before teaching Phases II, Steps 1 through 5. Continue to teach remaining phases and steps in the same manner.
2. Teacher may adjust the number of steps to correspond with situation in home or school.
3. *Caution:* This program requires modification by appropriate support personnel for use with students who have muscle tone problems, paralysis, or other physical handicaps.

SSS. Walks Down Stairs

Approximate Age for Skill Acquisition
21-60 months

TERMINAL OBJECTIVE:	Student walks down six steps without the handrail or the aid of the teacher's hands.
PREREQUISITE SKILLS:	Independent walking, creeps down stairs.
Phase I	Twenty-one months. Student walks down steps by holding on to hand rail with one hand and teacher's hand with the other hand, utilizing a walking kind of rhythm, wherein he moves one foot down the stairs and moves the other foot even with that foot before proceeding to the next step.
Phase II	Student walks down steps by holding on to handrail without the aid of teacher's hand and utilizing a walking type rhythm wherein he moves one foot down the stairs and moves the other foot even with that foot before proceeding to the next step.
Phase III	Twenty-five months. Student walks down steps without holding on to handrail and without aid of teacher's hand and utilizing a walking kind of rhythm wherein he moves one foot down the stairs and moves the other foot even with that foot before proceeding to the next step.
Phase IV	Thirty-six months. Student walks down steps by holding on to handrail with one hand and teacher's hand with the other hand, and alternating steps.
Phase V	Forty-three months. Student walks down steps by holding on to handrail without aid of teacher's hand and alternating steps.
Phase VI	Sixty months. Student walks down steps without the handrail or the aid of the teacher's hand.

The following steps are to be used with Phases I through VI:

Steps
-----

1. Two steps.
2. Three steps.
3. Four steps.
4. Five steps.
5. Six steps.

SUGGESTED MATERIALS: Flight of six steps, standard rise stairs.

TEACHING NOTES:
1. Teaching Sequence — Teach this skill beginning with Phase I, Step 1. Then teach Phase I, Steps 2 through 5 before teaching Phase II, Steps 1 through 5. Continue to teach remaining phases and steps in the same manner.
2. *Caution:* This program requires modification by appropriate support personnel for use with students who have muscle tone problems, paralysis, or other physical handicaps.

TTT. Picks Up Object From Floor — Standing

Approximate Age for Skill Acquisition 21-30 months

TERMINAL OBJECTIVE:	From a standing position, student leans over, picks up small lightweight object from floor, and returns to upright position without falling over.
PREREQUISITE SKILLS:	Ability to stand. Leans and regains balance, sitting. Protective extension forward and lateral. Ability to grasp.
Phase I	Student leans over and picks up object from a waist-level surface and regains standing without falling.
Phase II	Student leans over and picks up object from a hip-level surface and regains standing without falling.
Phase III	Student leans over and picks up object from a midthigh-level surface and regains standing without falling.
Phase IV	Student leans over and picks up object from a knee-level surface and regains standing without falling.
Phase V	Student leans over and picks up object from a midshin-level surface and regains standing without falling.
Phase VI	Student leans over and picks up object from an ankle-level surface and regains standing without falling.
Phase VII	From a standing position, student leans over, picks up small lightweight object from floor and returns to upright standing position without falling over.
SUGGESTED MATERIALS:	Surfaces that are appropriate for student's height, based on specifications in Phases I through VII. An adjustable table would be ideal.
TEACHING NOTES:	1. Teaching Sequence — Teach this skill be-

ginning with Phase I, then teach Phases II through VII.

2. *Caution:* This program requires modification by appropriate support personnel for use with students who have muscle tone problems, paralysis, or other physical handicaps.

UUU. Running

Approximate Age for
Skill Acquisition
24-48 months

TERMINAL OBJECTIVE: Student runs 300 yards in at least three minutes.

PREREQUISITE SKILLS: Independent walking.

Phase I — Student walks forward 25 yards at as rapid a pace as he can. Baseline is determined by averaging ten trials to get walking rate.

Phase II — Student moves forward 25 yards bearing own weight in running posture.

The following steps apply to Phase II only:

Steps
1. Reduce baseline time in Phase I (walking) by 10 percent.
2. Reduce baseline time in Phase I (walking) by 20 percent.
3. Reduce baseline time in Phase I (walking) by 30 percent.
4. Reduce baseline time in Phase I (walking) by 40 percent.
5. Reduce baseline time in Phase I (walking) by 50 percent.

Phase III — Student runs 50 yards, no time limit.
Phase IV — Student runs 100 yards, no time limit.
Phase V — Student runs 150 yards, no time limit.
Phase VI — Student runs 200 yards, no time limit.
Phase VII — Student runs 250 yards, no time limit.
Phase VIII — Student runs 300 yards.

The following steps are to be used with Phase VIII only:

Steps
1. Time of six minutes.
2. Time of five and one-half minutes.
3. Time of five minutes.
4. Time of four and one-half minutes.
5. Time of four minutes.
6. Time of three and one-half minutes.
7. Time of three minutes.

SUGGESTED MATERIALS: None.

TEACHING NOTES:
1. Teaching Sequence — Teach this skill beginning with Phase I. Then teach Phases II, Steps 1 through 5 before teaching Phases III through VII. Then teach Phase VIII, Steps 1 through 7.
2. The object of the program is to move the student from walking to running. The philosophy of Phase II, Steps 1 through 5 is based on the idea that a person should be able to run twice as fast as he walks. Phases III through VII extend the distance which the student is to run. Improving the student's running time should not be attempted until the 300-yard distance has been achieved.
3. If the student has difficulty mastering the running posture or increasing his speed, the teacher can branch the program to include having the teacher run along with the student. In this way she can also provide ongoing encouragement.
4. *Caution:* This program requires modification by appropriate support personnel for use with the students who have muscle tone problems, paralysis, or other physical handicaps.

VVV. Seats Self at Table Approximate Age for Skill Acquisition 2-3 years

TERMINAL OBJECTIVE:	Student seats self at appropriate-sized table, pulling chair and self up to table.
PREREQUISITE SKILLS:	Sitting, getting in and out of seat, standing.
Phase I	Student raises buttocks off chair seat, grasps seat, scoots chair forward until it reaches table with complete physical assistance provided by the teacher.
Phase II	Student raises buttocks off chair seat, grasps seat, scoots chair forward until it reaches table; teacher provides physical assistance to scoot student forward three-fourths of the way. Student completes task.
Phase III	Student raises buttocks off chair seat, grasps seat, scoots chair forward until it reaches table; teacher provides physical assistance to scoot student forward one-half of the way. Student completes task.
Phase IV	Student raises buttocks off chair seat, grasps seat, scoots chair forward until it reaches table; teacher provides physical assistance to scoot student forward one-fourth of the way. Student completes task.
Phase V	Student seats self at a table, pulling chair and self up to table.
SUGGESTED MATERIALS:	Table and chair appropriate to student's size.
TEACHING NOTES:	1. Teaching Sequence — Teach this skill beginning with Phase I. Then teach Phases II through V. 2. *Caution:* This program requires modification by appropriate support personnel for use with students who have muscle tone problems, paralysis, or other physical handicaps.

WWW. Rides Tricycle

Approximate Age for
Skill Acquisition
2-4 years

TERMINAL OBJECTIVE: Student rides tricycle, pushing down on pedals with feet alternately, for a distance of 50 feet in a forward and circular direction and for a distance of 5 feet backward.

PREREQUISITE SKILLS: Appropriate range of motion; sitting behavior; adequate strength in legs.

Phase I — Student rides tricycle in forward direction, feet held or taped on pedals. Teacher moves trike forward.

Phase II — Student rides tricycle in forward direction, feet held or taped on pedals. Teacher pushes down on knees in alternating pattern.

Phase III — Student rides in forward direction, feet held or taped on pedals. Teacher cues by tapping knees alternately.

Phase IV — Student rides tricycle in forward direction, feet held or taped on pedals.

Phase V — Student rides tricycle in forward direction, teacher holds feet on pedals by touching lightly.

Phase VI — Student rides tricycle in forward direction, keeping feet on pedals independently.

The following steps are to be used with Phases I through VI.

<u>Steps</u>
1. 2 feet.
2. 3 feet.
3. 4 feet.
4. 5 feet.
5. 10 feet.
6. 20 feet.
7. 30 feet.
8. 40 feet.
9. 50 feet.

Phase VII — Student rides tricycle in backward direction keeping feet on pedals. Teacher provides push on knees.

Phase VIII — Student rides tricycle in backward direction keeping feet on pedals.

The following steps are to be used *only* with Phases VII and VIII:

Steps
1. 2 feet.
2. 3 feet.
3. 4 feet.
4. 5 feet.

Phase IX   Student rides tricycle in 180° arc, keeping feet on pedals; teacher steers tricycle.

Phase X   Student rides tricycle in 180° arc, keeping feet on pedals. Student guides tricycle.

SUGGESTED MATERIALS: Tricycle appropriate for size of student.

TEACHING NOTES:
1. Teaching Sequence — Teach this skill beginning with Phase I, Step 1. Then teach Phase I, Steps 2 through 9 before teaching Phase II, Steps 1 through 9. Continue to teach Phases III through VI in the same manner. Teach Phase VII with Steps 1 through 4. Then teach Phases VIII, Steps 1 through 4, followed by Phases IX and X.
2. *Caution:* This program requires modification by appropriate support personnel for use with students who have muscle tone problems, paralysis, or other physical handicaps.

XXX. Jumps

Approximate Age of Skill Acquisition
3-5 years

TERMINAL OBJECTIVE: Student jumps up and down five times without assistance.

PREREQUISITE SKILLS: Standing on tiptoes.

Phase I — Student in crouching position on two-by-four board takes teacher's hands. Teacher completely assists child to jump off two-by-four board onto floor. Teacher jumps with student simultaneously (for model).

Phase II — Student, in crouching position on two-by-four board, takes teacher's hands. Teacher guides student up off two-by-four board and onto floor. To be correct, student must make some effort to jump. Teacher jumps with student simultaneously (for model).

Phase III — Student, in crouching position, takes both of teacher's hands and jumps up off floor. Teacher jumps with student simultaneously (for model).

Phase IV — Student, in crouching position, takes teacher's right hand and jumps up off floor. Teacher jumps with student simultaneously (for model).

Phase V — Student jumps up and down two times, resting one hand on teacher's arm. Teacher jumps with student simultaneously (for model).

Phase VI — Student jumps up and down three times, resting one hand on teacher's arm. Teacher jumps with student simultaneously (for model).

Phase VII — Student jumps up and down four times, resting one hand on teacher's arm. Teacher jumps with student simultaneously (for model).

Phase VIII — Student jumps up and down five times resting hand on teacher's arm. Teacher jumps with student simultaneously (for model).

Phase IX — Student jumps up and down five times without assistance.

SUGGESTED MATERIALS: Two-by-four board.

TEACHING NOTES:
1. Teaching Sequence — Teach this skill beginning with Phase I, then teach Phases II through IX.
2. A correct jump is one where both feet completely leave the floor surface.
3. *Caution:* This program requires modification by appropriate support personnel for use with students who have muscle tone problems, paralysis, or other physical handicaps.

YYY. Stands on Tiptoes with Eyes Open   Approximate Age for
                                                Skill Acquisition
                                                  4-6 years

Terminal Objective: Student stands on tiptoes with eyes open for five seconds.

Prerequisite Skills: Standing, grasping.

Phase I   Student extends arms above head and grasps broomstick with both hands.

Phase II   Student grasps broomstick with both hands and stands on tiptoes.

Phase III   Student grasps broomstick with dominant hand and stands on tiptoes.

Phase IV   Student grasps broomstick with four fingers of dominant hand and stands on tiptoes.

Phase V   Student grasps broomstick with index finger and middle finger and stands on tiptoes.

Phase VI   Student grasps broomstick with index finger and stands on tiptoes.

Phase VII   Student grasps broomstick with index finger and stands on toes, then releases. Student allowed to regrasp broomstick as needed to maintain balance.

Phase VIII   Student grasps broomstick with index finger and stands on toes, then releases. Maintains balance independently.

Phase IX   Student stands on tiptoes with eyes open.

The following steps are to be used with Phases I through IX:

Steps

1. Time of one second.
2. Time of two seconds.
3. Time of three seconds.
4. Time of four seconds.
5. Time of five seconds.

Suggested Materials: Broomstick or round-handled stick for grasping.

TEACHING NOTES:
1. Teaching Sequence — Teach this skill beginning with Phase I, Step 1. Then teach Phase I, Steps 2 through 5 before teaching Phase II, Steps 1 through 5. Continue to teach Phases III through VII in the same manner.
2. *Caution:* This program requires modification by appropriate support personnel for use with students who have muscle tone problems, paralysis, or other physical handicaps.

ZZZ. Walks Backward on a Line Approximate Age for Skill Acquisition 5-7 years

TERMINAL OBJECTIVE:	Student walks backward on a 1-inch-wide line for six steps by touching heel to toe along line without stepping off.
PREREQUISITE SKILLS:	Walking forward on a line.
Phase I	Student walks backward by touching heel to toe for one step without stepping off of a line 1 inch wide.
Phase II	Student walks backward by touching heel to toe for two steps without stepping off of a line 1 inch wide.
Phase III	Student walks backward by touching heel to toe for three steps without stepping off of a line 1 inch wide.
Phase IV	Student walks backward by touching heel to toe for four steps without stepping off of a line 1 inch wide.
Phase V	Student walks backward by touching heel to toe for five steps on a line 1 inch wide without stepping off.
Phase VI	Student walks backward by touching heel to toe for six steps along a line 1 inch wide without stepping off.
SUGGESTED MATERIALS:	Tape for marking line if necessary. A 1-inch line painted on a surface may also be used.
TEACHING NOTES:	1. Teaching Sequence — Teach this skill beginning with Phase 1. Then teach Phases II through VI. 2. *Caution:* This program requires modification by appropriate support personnel for use with students who have muscle tone problems, paralysis, or other physical handicaps.

AAAA. Stands on One Foot, Eyes Open   Approximate Age for
Skill Acquisition
5-6 years

TERMINAL OBJECTIVE:	Student stands on one leg for five seconds, other foot 3 inches off floor, eyes open and without assistance.
PREREQUISITE SKILLS:	Standing.
Phase I	Student stands facing wall with both hands on wall and lifts left foot 3 inches off floor with eyes open. Repeat for other side.
Phase II	Student stands facing wall with one hand on wall and lifts leg 3 inches off floor with eyes open. Repeat for other side.
Phase III	Student stands facing wall with four fingers on wall, left foot 3 inches off floor with eyes open. Repeat for other side.
Phase IV	Student stands facing wall with one index and one middle finger on wall, left foot 3 inches off floor with eyes open. Repeat for other side.
Phase V	Student stands facing wall with one index finger on wall, left leg 3 inches off floor with eyes open. Repeat for other side.
Phase VI	Student stands on right leg only, left foot 3 inches off floor, eyes open and without assistance. Repeat for other side.

The following steps are to be used with Phases I through VI:

Steps

1. Time of 1 second.
2. Time of 2 seconds.
3. Time of 3 seconds.
4. Time of 4 seconds.
5. Time of 5 seconds.

SUGGESTED MATERIALS:	Wall.
TEACHING NOTES:	1. Teaching Sequence — Teach this skill beginning with Phase I, Step 1. Then teach Phase I, Steps 2 through 5 before teaching

Phase II, Steps 1 through 5. Continue to teach remaining phases and steps in the same manner.
2. This sequence needs to be taught for each foot. Data should be maintained for the student's performance with each foot.
3. *Caution:* This program requires modification by appropriate support personnel for use with students who have muscle tone problems, paralysis, or other physical handicaps.

BBBB. Walks Forward on a Balance Beam Approximate Age for
Skill Acquisition
5-6 years

TERMINAL OBJECTIVE:	Student walks forward on a balance beam for a distance of 8 feet without stepping off.
PREREQUISITE SKILLS:	Walking.
Phase I	Student walks forward on 1-foot-square rubber mats placed in straight line.
Phase II	Student walks forward on 1-foot-square rubber mats staggered so that upper right-hand corner of one mat touches lower left hand corner of second mat and so on for eight mats.
Phase III	Student walks forward on 4-inch-wide tape line, placing heel of one foot against toe of other foot.
Phase IV	Student walks forward on 1-inch-wide straight line placing heel of one foot against toe of other foot.
Phase V	Student walks forward on two-by-four board placed on the floor.
Phase VI	Student walks forward on balance beam placed on the floor.
Phase VII	Student walks forward on balance beam raised 2 inches from floor.
Phase VIII	Student walks forward on balance beam raised 4 inches from floor.
Phase IX	Student walks forward on balance beam raised 6 inches from floor.

The following steps apply to each of the phases:

Steps

1. Distance of 1 foot without stepping off.
2. Distance of 2 feet without stepping off.
3. Distance of 3 feet without stepping off.
4. Distance of 4 feet without stepping off.

5. Distance of 5 feet without stepping off.
6. Distance of 6 feet without stepping off.
7. Distance of 7 feet without stepping off.
8. Distance of 8 feet without stepping off.

SUGGESTED MATERIALS: Tape for making line, square rubber mats, 8 foot two-by-four board, balance beam (four-by-four board, 8 feet long).

TEACHING NOTES:
1. Teaching Sequence — Teach this skill beginning with Phase I, Step 1. Then teach Phase I, Steps 2 through 8 before teaching Phase II, Steps 1 through 8. Teach remaining phases and steps in the same manner.
2. *Caution:* This program requires modification by appropriate support personnel for use with students who have muscle tone problems, paralysis or other physical handicaps.

CCCC. Stands Heel to Toe Approximate Age for
Skill Acquisition
5-6 years

TERMINAL OBJECTIVE:	Student stands in a heel to toe position with eyes closed.
PREREQUISITE SKILLS:	Standing.
Phase I	Student stands heel to toe with eyes open.
Phase II	Student stands heel to toe with eyes closed when teacher assists in placement, then releases when student is balanced. Student maintains momentarily.
Phase III	Student stands heel to toe with eyes closed.

The following steps are to be used with Phases I through III:

Steps

1. Student stands with feet next to each other, but with toe of left foot at a position halfway between heel and toe of right foot.
2. Student stands with feet next to each other, but with toe of left foot in a position directly behind the heel of right foot.
3. Student stands with his left toe touching the left part of his right heel.
4. Student stands with right foot placed directly in front of left foot so that heel of right foot touches toes of left foot.

SUGGESTED MATERIALS:	None.
TEACHING NOTES:	1. Teaching Sequence — Teach this skill beginning with Phase I, Step 1. Then teach Phase I, Steps 2 through 4 before teaching Phase II, Steps 1 through 4. Teach Phase III in the same manner.
	2. *Caution:* This program requires modification by appropriate support personnel for use with students who have muscle tone problems, paralysis, or other physical handicaps.

DDDD. Stands on Tiptoes, Eyes Closed

Approximate Age for Skill Acquisition
5-7 years

TERMINAL OBJECTIVE:	Student stands on tiptoes with eyes closed for five seconds.
PREREQUISITE SKILLS:	Standing on tiptoes, eyes open.
Phase I	Student grasps broomstick with both hands, and closes eyes.
Phase II	Student grasps broomstick with both hands, closes eyes, and stands on tiptoes.
Phase III	Student grasps broomstick with dominant hand, closes eyes, and stands on tiptoes.
Phase IV	Student grasps broomstick with four fingers of dominant hand, closes eyes, and stands on tiptoes.
Phase V	Student grasps broomstick with index and middle finger, closes eyes, and stands on tiptoes.
Phase VI	Student grasps broomstick with index finger and stands on tiptoes with eyes closed.
Phase VII	Student stands on tiptoes with eyes closed.

The following steps are to be used with Phases I through VII:

Steps

1. Time of one second.
2. Time of two seconds.
3. Time of three seconds.
4. Time of four seconds.
5. Time of five seconds.

SUGGESTED MATERIALS:	Broomstick or other round stick for grasping.
TEACHING NOTES:	1. Teaching Sequence — Teach this skill beginning with Phase I, Step 1. Then teach Phase I, Steps 2 through 5 before teaching Phase II, Steps 1 through 5. Continue to teach remaining phases and steps in the same manner.

2. *Caution:* This program requires modification by appropriate support personnel for use with students who have muscle tone problems, paralysis, or other physical handicaps.

EEEE. Stands on One Foot, Eyes Closed

Approximate Age for Skill Acquisition
5-7 years

TERMINAL OBJECTIVE:	Student stands on one leg only, with other foot 3 inches off floor, eyes closed and no assistance from teacher for five seconds.
PREREQUISITE SKILLS:	Standing on one foot with eyes open.
Phase I	Student stands facing wall with both hands on wall and lifts one foot 3 inches off floor with eyes closed. Repeat for other leg.
Phase II	Student stands facing wall with one hand on wall and lifts leg 3 inches off floor, eyes closed. Repeat for other leg.
Phase III	Student stands facing wall with four fingers on wall, one foot is 3 inches off floor, and eyes are closed. Repeat for other leg.
Phase IV	Student stands facing wall with one index and one middle finger on wall, one foot is 3 inches off floor, and eyes are closed. Repeat for other leg.
Phase V	Student stands facing wall with one index finger on wall, one leg is 3 inches off floor, and eyes are closed. Repeat for other leg.
Phase VI	Student stands on one leg only with other foot 3 inches off floor; eyes are closed and no assistance is given from teacher. Repeat for other leg.

The following steps are to be used with Phases I through VI:

Steps

1. Time of 1 second.
2. Time of 2 seconds.
3. Time of 3 seconds.
4. Time of 4 seconds.
5. Time of 5 seconds.

TEACHING NOTES:

1. Teaching Sequence — Teach this skill beginning with Phase I, Step 1. Then teach Phase I, Steps 2 through 5 before teaching

Phase II, Steps 1 through 5. Continue to teach remaining phases and steps in the same manner.

2. *Caution:* This program requires modification by appropriate support personnel for use with students who have muscle tone problems, paralysis, or other physical handicaps.

Chapter 4

FINE MOTOR SKILLS

THIS CHAPTER contains fine motor upper extremity sequences. Skills A through K are normally accomplished by nonhandicapped children during their first year of life. Skills L through P are second-year skills and skills Q through Y are third-year skills.

Before commencing any of these programs with students who exhibit physical anomalies, consultation should be sought with a physician and an appropriate medical support person, such as a physical therapist or an occupational therapist.

Seven of the sequences (A, D, E, G, H, J, K) require that the sequence be learned with each hand. A student should be taught each of these sequences with one hand before being taught the behavior with the other hand. In most instances, the student may not indicate a dominant hand; therefore, the teacher can arbitrarily choose which hand to teach first. If the student exhibits a dominant hand, the skill should be taught using the dominant hand before teaching the skill with the nondominant hand. Some teachers have found it easier to teach these behaviors for both hands concurrently. (This has not been our experience.) If that is the teacher's preference, separate data should be maintained for each hand.

Variations of Skills N, R, and S are frequently taught as prereading discrimination exercises. It is important to point out that the emphasis within this chapter is on motor skills and not on discrimination exercises.

As with other motor skills, some of the sequences in this section are reverse chained. (See Chapter 1 for a detailed description of reverse chaining.)

GLOSSARY

A glossary of terms relating to motor development, motion dysfunctions, and physical therapy is provided at the back of this volume.

FINE MOTOR SKILLS

SKILL	APPROXIMATE AGE FOR SKILL ACQUISITION
A. Maintains Grasp on Object — Supine	2-4 months
B. Brings Hands Together — Supine	2½-4 months
C. Reaches for Suspended Swinging Objects — Supine	3-5 months

D. Reaches for Object — Prone	4-5	months
E. Reaches for and Picks Up, Using Whole Hand Grasp	5-6	months
F. Grasps Object with Both Hands	5-7	months
G. Intentionally Releases Object from Grasp	5-8	months
H. Transfers Object from One Hand to the Other	5-8	months
I. Grasps Two Objects, One in Each Hand	7-10	months
J. Reaches for and Picks Up Object, Using Thumb/Fingertips Grasp	7½-12	months
K. Picks Up and Grasps Object, Using Neat Pincer Grasp (Thumb and Index Finger)	7-12	months
L. Puts Objects in Small-Mouthed Container	10-14	months
M. Moves Object from One Container to Another	16-18	months
N. Puts Rings on a Peg	15-17	months
O. Builds a Tower	15-21	months
P. Turns Knob	1½-21	years
Q. Turns Pages of a Book, One at a Time	2-2½	years
R. Puts Cylinders in Same-Sized Receptacle	2-3	years
S. Puts Pegs in Pegboard	2-3½	years
T. Strings Beads	2-3½	years
U. Unscrews and Screws on Jar Lid	2½-3½	years
V. Pastes Paper	2½-3½	years
W. Uses Tongs to Pick Up Objects	2½-3½	years
X. Cuts with Scissors	2½-3½	years
Y. Laces Ten-Hole Card	3-4	years

Fine Motor Skills

A. Maintains Grasp on Object — Supine

Approximate Age for Skill Acquisition
2-4 months

TERMINAL OBJECTIVE:	In supine position, student will maintain grasp on object for five seconds when it is placed in hand. Task should be completed for each hand separately.
PREREQUISITE SKILLS:	Appropriate range of motion of fingers.
Phase I	When object is placed in student's hand, teacher gives complete physical assistance for student to grasp object for one second.
Phase II	When object is placed in student's hand, teacher gives initial physical assistance for student to grasp object, student maintains grasp for one second.
Phase III	When object is placed in student's hand, teacher gives light squeeze to initiate grasp; student maintains grasp for one second.
Phase IV	When object is placed in student's hand, student grasps and maintains.

The following steps are to be used with Phase IV only:

Steps

1. One second.
2. Two seconds.
3. Three seconds.
4. Four seconds.
5. Five seconds.

SUGGESTED MATERIALS:	An object that is easy to grasp, such as rattle. *Important:* Object should be large enough so student will not swallow it.
TEACHING NOTES:	1. Teaching Sequence — Teach this skill beginning with Phase I. Then teach Phases II through III before teaching Phase IV, Steps 1 through 5.
	2. This task should be taught for one hand first. After the student learns the tasks with

one hand, teach the behaviors for the other hand.
3. Student may want to mouth the object after grasping it. This is a normal method of exploration and should not be discouraged.
4. *Caution:* This program requires modification by appropriate support personnel for use with children with muscle tone problems or paralysis.

B. Brings Hands Together — Supine

Approximate Age for Skill Acquisition
2½-4 months

TERMINAL OBJECTIVE:	In supine position, student will bring hands together at midline and will maintain and touch/explore hands for five seconds.
PREREQUISITE SKILLS:	Student has exhibited range of motion required.
Phase I	Student brings hands together with complete physical assistance from teacher. Teacher assists student to touch all hand surfaces (if necessary) for five seconds.
Phase II	Student brings hands together with physical assistance from teacher at wrists. Teacher assists student to touch all hand surfaces (if necessary) for five seconds.
Phase III	Student brings hands together with physical assistance at forearms from teacher. Teacher assists student to touch all hand surfaces (if necessary) for five seconds.
Phase IV	Student brings hands together with physical assistance from teacher at shoulders. Teacher assists student to touch all hand surfaces (if necessary) for five seconds.
Phase V	Student brings hands together and touches and explores hands.

The following steps are to be used with Phase V only:

Steps

1. One second.
2. Two seconds.
3. Three seconds.
4. Four seconds.
5. Five seconds.

SUGGESTED MATERIALS: Pudding, tape loop, hand cream, Slime® (see Teaching Note #4).

TEACHING NOTES: 1. Teaching Sequence — Teach this skill be-

ginning with Phase I. Then teach Phases II through IV before going to Phase V, Steps 1 through 5.
2. This behavior is taught with student in supine position.
3. Student should touch and explore hands rather than simply hold them in one position for the full five seconds.
4. For placement testing the terminal objective, one of the suggested materials may be placed on the student's hands to provide incentive for the behavior. Do not use toxic materials if the student tends to mouth everything. The tactile materials suggested may also be used as a branch alternative.
5. *Caution:* The program requires modification by appropriate support personnel for use with students with muscle tone problems or paralysis.

C. Reaches for Suspended Swinging Object — Supine

Approximate Age for Skill Acquisition
3-5 months

TERMINAL OBJECTIVE:	Student in supine position reaches for suspended swinging object with one or both hands when it is presented within the field of vision, responding within two seconds.
PREREQUISITE SKILLS:	Ability to focus on an object that is suspended and swinging.
Phase I	Student reaches for suspended, swinging object that is presented within the field of vision, given complete physical assistance.
Phase II	Student reaches for suspended, swinging object that is presented within the field of vision, given push halfway in direction of object.
Phase III	Student reaches for suspended, swinging object when it is presented within the field of vision, given initial light touch to initiate movement in direction of object.
Phase IV	Student reaches for suspended, swinging object when it is presented within the field of vision, responding within thirty seconds.
Phase V	Student reaches for suspended, swinging object when it is presented within the field of vision, responding within twenty seconds.
Phase VI	Student reaches for suspended, swinging object when it is presented within the field of vision, responding within ten seconds.
Phase VII	Student reaches for suspended, swinging object when it is presented within the field of vision, responding within five seconds.
Phase VIII	Student reaches for suspended, swinging object when it is presented within the field of vision, responding within two seconds.
SUGGESTED MATERIALS:	Any object that is reinforcing to the student, suspended with string or yarn. Object may need to be changed frequently.

TEACHING NOTES:
1. Teaching Sequence — Teach Phases I through VIII in order.
2. This program is taught from the supine position.
3. Reach with one or both hands is acceptable.
4. It will be necessary for the teacher to establish the student's field of vision prior to starting this program.
5. *Caution:* This program requires modification by appropriate support personnel for use with children with muscle tone problems or paralysis.

D. Reaches for Objects — Prone

Approximate Age for
Skill Acquisition
4-5 months

TERMINAL OBJECTIVE:	Student reaches for and touches object with hands/arms while in prone position. Task should be completed for each hand separately.
PREREQUISITE SKILLS:	Ability to bear weight on elbows; ability to shift weight from one arm to the other. Student has demonstrated head control in prone position.
Phase I	In prone position, student reaches for object with hand/arm, given complete physical assistance by the teacher, who moves student's arm in direction of object.
Phase II	In prone position, student reaches for object with hand/arm, given physical assistance by the teacher, who touches student's arm to initiate reaching. Student reaches and touches object.
Phase III	In prone position, student reaches for and touches object with hand/arm.
SUGGESTED MATERIALS:	Any object that appeals to or is known to be highly reinforcing to student.
TEACHING NOTES:	1. Teaching Sequence — Teach Phases I through III in order. 2. Although grasping the object is not required for this task to be correct, score correct if student grasps object after reaching. 3. Object is placed within easy reaching distance of student's hand, forward of head 6 inches and to the side of head corresponding to grasping hand. 4. This behavior should be taught for one hand first. After the student learns the behavior with one hand, teach the behavior for the other hand. 5. *Caution:* This program requires modification by appropriate support personnel for use with children with muscle tone problems or paralysis.

E. Reaches for and Picks Up, Using Whole Hand Grasp

Approximate Age for Skill Acquisition
5-6 months

TERMINAL OBJECTIVE: Student reaches for and picks up object, using whole hand grasp. Task should be completed for each hand separately.

PREREQUISITE SKILLS: Appropriate range of motion; maintains grasp on object.

Phase I — Student's hand is guided with complete physical assistance to object; student picks up object, using whole hand grasp.

Phase II — Student's hand is guided to object; student picks up object, using whole hand grasp, given complete physical assistance.

Phase III — Student's hand is guided to object and placed in grasping position around it; student picks up object, using whole hand grasp.

Phase IV — Student's hand is guided to object; student picks up object, using whole hand grasp.

Phase V — Student's hand is guided halfway toward object; student picks up object, using whole hand grasp.

Phase VI — Student's hand is guided one fourth of the way toward object; student picks up object using whole hand grasp.

Phase VII — Teacher gives student's hand initial push toward object; student picks up object, using whole hand grasp.

Phase VIII — Student reaches for and picks up objects, using whole hand grasp.

SUGGESTED MATERIALS: Toy or object that appeals to or is known to be highly reinforcing to the student. Object should be approximately 1 inch in diameter.

TEACHING NOTES:
1. Teaching Sequence — Teach Phases I through VIII in order.
2. This behavior should be taught from a sitting position.

3. Teacher places object within student's reach.
4. This task should be taught for one hand first. After the student learns the behavior with one hand, teach the behavior for the other hand.
5. Student may want to mouth the object after grasping it. This is a normal method of exploration and should not be discouraged.
6. *Caution:* This program requires modification by appropriate support personnel for use with children with muscle tone problems or paralysis.

F. Grasps Object with Both Hands

Approximate Age for Skill Acquisition
5-7 months

TERMINAL OBJECTIVE:	Student grasps object with both hands simultaneously for five seconds from a supine or sitting position.
PREREQUISITE SKILLS:	Appropriate range of motion. Student has demonstrated reaching motion. Student can grasp object with one hand (whole hand grasp).
Phase I	Student grasps object with both hands with teacher holding student's hands around object.
Phase II	Student grasps object with both hands; teacher initiates holding, releases assistance, and student maintains grasp.
Phase III	Student grasps object with both hands and holds.

The following steps are to be used with Phases II and III only:

Steps
1. One second.
2. Two seconds.
3. Three seconds.
4. Four seconds.
5. Five seconds.

SUGGESTED MATERIALS: Large toy or object that appeals to or is known to be reinforcing to the student. Object should be large enough so student *cannot* grasp in one hand.

TEACHING NOTES:
1. Teaching Sequence — Teach this skill beginning with Phase I. Then teach Phase II, Steps 1 through 5 before Phase III, Steps 1 through 5.
2. Student should be in a sitting or supine position and object should be presented at midline.
3. Student may want to mouth the object after grasping. This is a normal method of exploration and should not be discouraged.

4. *Caution:* This program requires modification by appropriate support personnel for use with children with muscle tone problems or paralysis.

G. Intentionally Releases Object from Grasp

Approximate Age for Skill Acquisition
5-8 months

TERMINAL OBJECTIVE:	Student releases object by letting go completely.
PREREQUISITE SKILLS:	Whole hand grasp.
Phase I	Given verbal cue, student releases object when teacher bends hand at wrist by pushing on back of student's hand.
Phase II	Given verbal cue, student releases object when teacher taps back of student's hand.
Phase III	Given verbal cue, student releases object.
SUGGESTED MATERIALS:	Object or toy should be appropriate size for student's hand.
TEACHING NOTES:	1. Teaching Sequence — Teach Phases I through III in order. 2. This program may be conducted in supine or sitting position. 3. This program should be conducted with one hand. After learning the behavior with one hand, the student should be taught the behavior for the other hand. 4. *Caution:* This program requires modification by appropriate support personnel for use with children with muscle tone problems or paralysis.

Fine Motor Skills

H. Transfers Object from One Hand to the Other

Approximate Age for Skill Acquisition
5-8 months

TERMINAL OBJECTIVE: When object is placed in student's hand, student independently moves hand to opposite side, places object in opposite hand, and releases.

PREREQUISITE SKILLS: Ability to grasp an object with whole hand grasp; appropriate range of motion; ability to release an object; ability to bring hands together.

Phase I — When object is placed in student's hand, teacher assists student to move hand to opposite side, to place object in opposite hand, and to release.

Phase II — When object is placed in student's hand, teacher assists student to move hand to opposite side and to place object in opposite hand. Student releases object.

Phase III — When object is placed in student's hand, teacher assists student to move hand to opposite side. Student places object in opposite hand and releases.

Phase IV — When object is placed in student's hand, teacher prompts student with touch to move hand to opposite side. Student places object in opposite hand and releases.

Phase V — When object is placed in student's hand, student independently moves hand to opposite side, places object in opposite hand and releases.

SUGGESTED MATERIALS: Small toy or object, appropriate to size of student's hand.

TEACHING NOTES:
1. Teaching Sequence — Teach Phases I through V in order.
2. This program should be taught for one hand before teaching it for the other hand.
3. This program should preferably be taught

in the sitting position. However, if the student is unable to sit, the program can be taught with the student in the supine position.
4. *Caution:* This program requires modification by appropriate support personnel for use with students with muscle tone problems or paralysis.

Fine Motor Skills 219

I. Grasps Two Objects, One in Each Hand

Approximate Age for Skill Acquisition
7-10 months

TERMINAL OBJECTIVE:	Student grasps two objects, one in each hand and maintains grasp for five seconds.
PREREQUISITE SKILLS:	Whole hand grasping ability with each hand; appropriate range of motion.
Phase I	Student's hands are placed on objects. Teacher assists student to grasp and hold.
Phase II	Student grasps objects, one in each hand when placed; teacher assists student to hold objects.
Phase III	Student grasps objects, one in each hand when placed; teacher initiates holding then releases, and student maintains hold on objects.
Phase IV	Student grasps and holds two objects, one in each hand, with teacher physically prompting by touching student's hands.
Phase V	Student grasps and holds two objects, one in each hand.

The following steps are to be used with Phases III through V:

Steps

1. One second.
2. Two seconds.
3. Three seconds.
4. Four seconds.
5. Five seconds.

SUGGESTED MATERIALS:	Small objects such as blocks or beads.
TEACHING NOTES:	1. Teaching Sequence — Teach this skill beginning with Phases I and II. Then teach Phase III, Steps 1 through 5 before teaching Phase IV, Steps 1 through 5 and Phase V, Steps 1 through 5.
	2. Student is likely to bang objects together. This is normal and should not be restrained for this program.
	3. Student may want to mouth the objects after

grasping them. This is a normal method of exploration and should not be discouraged.
4. *Caution:* This program requires modification by appropriate support personnel for use with children with muscle tone problems or paralysis.

J. Reaches for and Picks Up Object, Using Thumb/Fingertips Grasp

Approximate Age for Skill Acquisition 7½-12 months

TERMINAL OBJECTIVE:	Student reaches for and grasps an object, using thumb/fingertips grasp. Task should be completed for each hand separately.
PREREQUISITE SKILLS:	Student has demonstrated whole hand grasping ability.
Phase I	Student's hand is guided to object with complete physical assistance. Student is assisted to pick up object using thumb/fingertips grasp.
Phase II	Student's hand is guided to object. Student is assisted to pick up objects using thumb/fingertips grasp. Teacher releases, and student maintains grasp.
Phase III	Student's hand is guided to object. Teacher holds student's wrist 2 to 3 inches off table so that student must grasp object with fingertips.
Phase IV	Student's hand is guided to object. Teacher touches under wrist so that student must grasp object with fingertips.
Phase V	Student's hand is guided to object. Teacher releases and student picks up object using thumb/fingertips grasp.
Phase VI	Student's hand is guided three-fourths of the way toward object. Student picks up object using thumb/fingertips grasp.
Phase VII	Student's hand is guided halfway toward object. Student picks up object using thumb/fingertips grasp.
Phase VIII	Student's hand is guided one-fourth of the way toward object. Student picks up object using thumb/fingertips grasp.
Phase IX	Teacher gives student's hand initial push towards object. Student picks up object using thumb/fingertips grasp.
Phase X	Student reaches for and picks up object using thumb/fingertips grasp.

The following steps are to be used for **Phase X** *only:*

Steps
1. 1-inch cube or similar size object or food.
2. ¾-inch cube or dowel, or similar size object or food.
3. ½-inch cube or dowel, or similar size object or food.
4. Raisin-size object.

SUGGESTED MATERIALS: Small block or toy, finger foods, or any object that appeals to or is known to be highly reinforcing to student. For Phases I through IX use an object approximately 1-inch in size. For Phase X see steps.

TEACHING NOTES:
1. Teaching Sequence — Teach Phase I followed by Phases II through IX. Then teach Phase X, Steps 1 through 4.
2. This behavior should be taught for one hand first. After student learns this behavior for one hand, it should be taught for the other hand.
3. Teacher should be careful to place object within student's reach.
4. *Caution:* This program requires modification by appropriate support personnel for use with students with muscle tone problems or paralysis.

Fine Motor Skills

K. Picks Up and Grasps Object, Using Neat Pincer Grasp (Thumb and Index Finger)

Approximate Age for Skill Acquisition
7-12 months

TERMINAL OBJECTIVE:	Student picks up and grasps object for five seconds, using neat pincer grasp.
PREREQUISITE SKILLS:	Appropriate range of motion; student demonstrates thumb/fingertips grasp.
Phase I	Teacher opens student's hand, places object against index finger, and assists student to grasp object with thumb and index finger.
Phase II	Teacher opens student's hand, places object against index finger, and assists student to grasp object with thumb and index finger. Student maintains grasp independently.

The following steps are to be used with Phase II only:

Steps

1. One second.
2. Two seconds.
3. Three seconds.
4. Four seconds.
5. Five seconds.

Phase III	Teacher opens student's hand, places object against index finger, and gives student five seconds to independently place thumb and index finger together. Student maintains grasp for five seconds.
Phase IV	Student opens hand; teacher places object against index finger and gives student five seconds to independently place thumb and index finger together. Student maintains grasp for five seconds.
Phase V	Student picks up object, using thumb and index finger, and maintains grasp for five seconds.
SUGGESTED MATERIALS:	Small bead, small peg, raisin, other foods, such as cereals, small marshmallows, grapes, etc. (½ inch in diameter or less).

TEACHING NOTES:
1. Teaching Sequence — Teach this skill beginning with Phase I. Then teach Phase II, Steps 1 through 5 before going to Phases III through V.
2. Teacher holds object in place on student's index finger until student grasps, for all phases, except Phase V.
3. This task should be taught for one hand first. After the student learns the task with one hand, teach the behavior for the other hand.
4. *Caution:* This program requires modification by appropriate support personnel for use with students with muscle tone problems or paralysis.

L. Puts Objects in Small-Mouthed Container Approximate Age for Skill Acquisition 10-14 months

TERMINAL OBJECTIVE:	Student puts two clothespins in container with 2-inch diameter mouth.
PREREQUISITE SKILLS:	Ability to grasp and release objects; appropriate range of motion.
Phase I	Student is given complete physical assistance by teacher to bring hand over container. Student drops block in a 6-inch container.
Phase II	Student is given physical assistance by teacher to bring hand three-fourths of the way to container. Student puts block in a 6-inch container.
Phase III	Student is given physical assistance by teacher to bring hand one-half of the way to container. Student puts block in a 6-inch container.
Phase IV	Student is given physical assistance by teacher to bring hand one-fourth of the way to container. Student puts block in a 6-inch container.
Phase V	Student brings hand to container and puts object(s) in container independently.

The following steps are to be used with Phase V only:

Steps

1. Student puts one block in container with 6-inch diameter mouth.
2. Student puts two blocks in container with 6-inch diameter mouth.
3. Student puts one block in container with 4-inch diameter mouth.
4. Student puts two blocks in container with 4-inch diameter mouth.
5. Student puts one clothespin in container with 2-inch diameter mouth.
6. Student puts two clothespins in container with 2-inch diameter mouth.

SUGGESTED MATERIALS: 1-inch cube blocks, clothespins, containers (one each) with 6-inch, 4-inch, and 2-inch diameter mouths.
Important: Use masking tape or protective covering to conceal sharp edges if metal cans are used.

TEACHING NOTES: 1. Teaching Sequence — Teach this skill beginning with Phase I. Then teach Phases II through IV, then teach Phase V, Steps 1 through 6.

M. Moves Object From One Container to Another

Approximate Age for Skill Acquisition
16-18 months

TERMINAL OBJECTIVE:	Student removes object from one container and places it in second container.
PREREQUISITE SKILLS:	Ability to grasp and release an object. Appropriate range of motion.
Phase I	Teacher guides student's hand to first container and assists student to take object from container. Teacher guides hand to second container; student releases object.
Phase II	Teacher guides student's hand to first container and assists student to take object from container. Teacher guides hand halfway to second container; student places object in second container.
Phase III	Teacher guides student's hand to first container and assists student to take object from container. Student moves object to second container and releases.
Phase IV	Teacher guides student's hand to first container. Student takes object from container, moves hand to second container, and releases object.
Phase V	Student moves hand to first container, takes object, moves hand to second container, and releases object.
SUGGESTED MATERIALS:	1-inch cube blocks or other small objects, and two containers with 6-inch diameter mouths. A shallow box or clear deep container is desirable so that student can see object readily. *Important:* Use masking tape or protective covering to conceal sharp edges if metal cans are used.
TEACHING NOTES:	1. Teaching Sequence — Teach Phases I through V in order.

N. Puts Rings on a Peg

Approximate Age for
Skill Acquisition
15-17 months

TERMINAL OBJECTIVE: Student puts five rings on a peg. (For the task to be considered correct, it is not necessary that rings be put on in any particular order.)

PREREQUISITE SKILLS: Ability to grasp and release objects; appropriate range of motion.

Phase I — Teacher physically assists student to put one ring on peg.

Phase II — Teacher guides student at forearm to put one ring on peg.

Phase III — Student puts one ring on peg.

Phase IV — Student puts two rings on peg.

Phase V — Student puts three rings on peg.

Phase VI — Student puts four rings on peg.

Phase VII — Student puts five rings on peg.

SUGGESTED MATERIALS: Five rings of same size and a 1-inch diameter peg. Graduated rings may be used but may be placed on peg in any order.

TEACHING NOTES:
1. Teaching Sequence — Teach Phases I through VII in order.
2. If student has difficulty putting rings on a 1 inch diameter peg, use rings with 2-inch diameter openings and continue to use the 1-inch diameter peg. After the student has learned the skill using rings with larger openings, the skill can be taught using rings with 1-inch diameter openings.

Fine Motor Skills

O. Builds a Tower

Approximate Age for
Skill Acquisition
15-21 months

TERMINAL OBJECTIVE: Student builds a tower of five blocks placed in a vertical direction.

PREREQUISITE SKILLS: Ability to grasp and release objects; appropriate range of motion.

Phase I — Fifteen months. Teacher gives student complete assistance to pick up one cube and place on one other cube for a tower of two, using 4 by 4 inch blocks.

Phase II — Fifteen months. Student picks up cube, and teacher assists student to place cube on one other cube for a tower of two, using 4 by 4 inch blocks.

Phase III — Fifteen to sixteen months. Student builds tower of two by stacking one cube on one other cube vertically, using 4 by 4 inch blocks.

Phase IV — Fifteen to sixteen months. Student builds tower of two by stacking one cube on one other cube vertically.

Phase V — Sixteen to twenty-one months. Student builds tower by stacking three cubes vertically.

Phase VI — Sixteen to twenty-one months. Student builds tower by stacking four cubes vertically.

Phase VII — Sixteen months. Student builds tower by stacking five cubes vertically.

The following steps are to be used with Phases IV through VII:

Steps

1. Medium-sized blocks measuring 2 by 2 inches.
2. Small blocks measuring 1 by 1 inch.

SUGGESTED MATERIALS: Two 4 by 4 inch blocks, five 2 by 2 inch blocks, and five 1 by 1 inch blocks.

TEACHING NOTES:
1. Teaching Sequence — Teach this skill beginning with Phase I. Then teach Phases II and III, before teaching Phases IV through

VII, Step 1. Then teach Phases IV through VII, Step 2.
2. Note the age norms that correspond to phases.
3. Procedure — For Phases I through III, which teach the student to stack one cube on another using large blocks, only place two blocks on the table. Similarly, for Phases IV, V, VI, and VII place only two, three, four, and five blocks respectively in front of the student. In this way, when all the blocks are stacked, he will know he is finished with the tower.

P. Turns Knob

Approximate Age for Skill Acquisition
1½-2 years

TERMINAL OBJECTIVE:	Student turns knob in clockwise direction.
PREREQUISITE SKILLS:	Whole hand grasp (Step 1) thumb/fingertips or pincer grasp (Step 2); appropriate range of motion.
Phase I	Student holds knob with fingers (and palm of hand for Step 1).
Phase II	Student makes one turn of knob, clockwise, teacher giving complete physical assistance.
Phase III	Student makes one turn of knob clockwise, assistance given for first half of the way around.
Phase IV	Student makes one turn of knob independently.

The following steps are to be used with Phases I through IV:

<u>Steps</u>
1. Large knob, 2 inches in diameter.
2. Medium knob, 1 inch in diameter.

SUGGESTED MATERIALS:	Toy radio or music box knobs, 1 and 2 inches in diameter; free-turning doorknob.
TEACHING NOTES:	1. Teaching Sequence — Teach this skill beginning with Phase I, Step 1. Then teach Phases II through IV, Step 1. Then teach Phases I through IV, Step 2.
	2. This sequence may be adapted for teaching the student to turn any kind of knob. For instance, to teach the student to open a door, add Phase V, "Student pulls door open."

Q. Turns Pages of a Book, One at a Time Approximate Age for Skill Acquisition 2-2½ years

TERMINAL OBJECTIVE:	Student opens book, turns five pages one by one, from front to back.
PREREQUISITE SKILLS:	Pincer grasp; appropriate range of motion.
Phase I	Student opens book.
Phase II	Student opens and closes book.
Phase III	Student opens book, turns any number of pages together once.
Phase IV	Student opens book, turns one page, teacher giving complete physical assistance.
Phase V	Student opens book, turns one page, teacher placing student's hand on page; student turns it alone.
Phase VI	Student opens book, turns five pages, one by one, from front to back.

The following steps are to be used with Phases I through VI:

<u>Steps</u>

1. Toddler book with thick cardboard pages.
2. Cloth book.
3. Regular book.

SUGGESTED MATERIALS:	Toddler book with thick cardboard pages, book with cloth pages, and regular book with paper pages.
TEACHING NOTES:	1. Teaching Sequence — Teach this skill beginning with Phase I, Step 1. Then teach Phases II through VI, Step 1 before teaching Phases I through VI, Step 2. Continue to teach remaining phases and steps in same manner.

R. Puts Cylinders in Same-Sized Receptacle Approximate Age for
Skill Acquisition
2-3 years

TERMINAL OBJECTIVE:	Student puts ten cylinders in ten same-sized receptacles. (For task to be considered correct, it is not necessary that cylinders be put in receptacles in any particular order.)
PREREQUISITE SKILLS:	Ability to grasp with thumb and fingers; appropriate range of motion.
Phase I	Teacher guides student to put one cylinder in receptacle.
Phase II	Teacher guides student to place one cylinder over receptacle. Student puts cylinder in receptacle.
Phase III	Student puts one cylinder in receptacle.
Phase IV	Student puts two cylinders in two receptacles.
Phase V	Student puts three cylinders in three receptacles.
Phase VI	Student puts four cylinders in four receptacles.
Phase VII	Student puts five cylinders in five receptacles.
Phase VIII	Student puts six cylinders in six receptacles.
Phase IX	Student puts seven cylinders in seven receptacles.
Phase X	Student puts eight cylinders in eight receptacles.
Phase XI	Student puts nine cylinders in nine receptacles.
Phase XII	Student puts ten cylinders in ten receptacles.
SUGGESTED MATERIALS:	Long wooden unit with ten same-sized receptacles and ten same-sized cylinders with handles or knobs.
TEACHING NOTES:	1. Teaching Sequence — Teach Phases I through XII in order.

S. Puts Pegs in Pegboard

Approximate Age for Skill Acquisition
2-3½ years

TERMINAL OBJECTIVE:	Student puts five short, shouldered pegs in the holes of small wooden or plastic pegboard.
PREREQUISITE SKILLS:	Ability to pick up objects and grasp with a neat pincer grasp (thumb and index finger).
Phase I	Teacher physically assists student to put one peg in hole of rubber pegboard.
Phase II	Teacher assists student to place one peg over hole in rubber pegboard. Student pushes peg into the hole.
Phase III	Student puts large pegs in the holes of a rubber pegboard independently.
Phase IV	Student puts tall, slim pegs in the holes of a large wooden or plastic pegboard independently.
Phase V	Student puts short pegs in the holes of a small wooden or plastic pegboard independently.

The following steps are to be used with Phases III through V only:

<u>Steps</u>

1. Student puts one peg in hole.
2. Student puts two pegs in hole.
3. Student puts three pegs in hole.
4. Student puts four pegs in hole.
5. Student puts five pegs in hole.

SUGGESTED MATERIALS:

Phase I-III

2-inch plastic shouldered pegs with rubber pegboard.

Phase IV

2-inch tall round wooden pegs with wooden pegboard.

Phase V

½-inch tall wooden shouldered pegs with wooden pegboard.

Teaching Notes:

1. Teaching Sequence — Teach this skill beginning with Phase I, then teach Phase II. Then teach Phase III, Steps 1 through 5 before teaching Phase IV, Steps 1 through 5 and Phase V, Steps 1 through 5.
2. Pegs can be placed in holes to form any pattern. They do not need to be placed in a line.

T. Strings Beads

Approximate Age for Skill Acquisition
2-3½ years

TERMINAL OBJECTIVE:	Student strings five beads by holding bead, inserting lace into hole, pushing lace through, moving bead to other hand, and pulling bead to end of lace.
PREREQUISITE SKILLS:	Neat pincer grasp (thumb and index finger).
Phase I	With tip of string through the bead, student pulls tip end so that bead is all the way to end of string.
Phase II	Student holds bead with one hand with tip of string at edge of hole and pulls string with the other so that bead is all the way to the end of string.
Phase III	Student holds bead, pushes lace final one-half of the way through bead, moves bead to other hand, and pulls bead to end of string.
Phase IV	Student holds bead, pushes lace through bead when tip is placed at hole, moves bead to other hand, and pulls bead to end of string.
Phase V	Student holds bead, inserts lace into hole, pushes lace through, moves bead to other hand, and pulls bead to end of lace.

The following steps are to be used with Phases I through V:

Steps

1. Student strings one bead.   — Phases I through V
2. Student strings two beads.   ⎫
3. Student strings three beads. ⎬ Phase V only
4. Student strings four beads. ⎪
5. Student strings five beads. ⎭

SUGGESTED MATERIALS:	Jumbo wooden beads 1- to 1½-inch diameter, string with tip at least ¼-inch longer than bead hole and about 1 foot long — by Playskool®.
TEACHING NOTES:	1. Teaching Sequence — Teach this skill beginning with Phase I, Step 1 before teaching Phase II through V, Step 1. Then teach Phase V, Steps 2 through 5.

U. Unscrews and Screws on Jar Lid

Approximate Age for Skill Acquisition
2½-3½ years

TERMINAL OBJECTIVE:	Student unscrews and screws a jar lid 4 inches in diameter.
PREREQUISITE SKILLS:	Ability to grasp jar with nondominant hand and grasp jar lid with dominant hand.
Phase I	Student unscrews jar lid given complete physical assistance by teacher.
Phase II	Student unscrews jar lid three-fourths of the way with physical assistance by teacher and final one-fourth of the way unassisted.
Phase III	Student unscrews jar lid halfway with physical assistance by teacher and final halfway unassisted.
Phase IV	Student unscrews jar lid one-fourth of the way with physical assistance by teacher and final three-fourths of the way unassisted.
Phase V	Student unscrews jar lid.
Phase VI	Student screws jar lid given complete physical assistance by teacher.
Phase VII	Student screws jar lid three-fourths of the way given physical assistance by teacher and final one-fourth of the way unassisted.
Phase VIII	Student screws jar lid halfway with physical assistance by the teacher and final halfway unassisted.
Phase IX	Student screws jar lid one-fourth of the way with physical assistance by teacher and final three-fourths of the way unassisted.
Phase X	Student screws jar lid.
Phase XI	Student unscrews and screws a jar lid.

The following steps apply to Phase XI:

Steps

1. 2-inch diameter lid.
2. 3-inch diameter lid.
3. 4-inch diameter lid.

SUGGESTED MATERIALS: Jars with approximately 2-inch, 3-inch, and 4-inch diameter lids. Jars should be small enough to easily fit in student's hand. For Phases I through X, use the 2-inch diameter lid.

TEACHING NOTES:
1. Teaching Sequence — Teach Phase I, then Phases II through X before teaching Phase XI, Steps 1, 2, and 3.
2. Student may use both hands if lid is too large to grasp with one hand.
3. To make this activity more interesting, use a clear jar and put a reward inside.

V. Pastes Paper

Approximate Age for
Skill Acquisition
2½–3½ years

TERMINAL OBJECTIVE: Student pastes 3-inch diameter circle of paper on circle form that has ⅛-inch wider boundary.

PREREQUISITE SKILLS: Neat pincer grasp (thumb and index finger).

Phase I — Student pats pasted piece of paper in place.

Phase II — Student picks up pasted piece of paper and pats paper in place.

Phase III — Student smears paste on piece of paper, picks it up, and pats in place.

Phase IV — Student places drop of paste on piece of paper, smears, picks up, and pats in place.

Phase V — Student pastes 2-inch wide straight strip of paper in place.

Phase VI — Student pastes 3-inch diameter circle of paper in place.

The following steps are to be used with Phases V through VI:

Steps

1. Paper pasted on form with boundaries 2 inches wider than piece to be pasted.
2. Paper pasted on form with boundaries 1 inch wider than piece to be pasted.
3. Paper pasted on form with boundaries ½ inch wider than piece to be pasted.
4. Paper pasted on form with boundaries ¼ inch wider than piece to be pasted.
5. Paper pasted on form with boundaries ⅛ inch wider than piece to be pasted.

SUGGESTED MATERIALS: Use heavy paper such as construction paper.

TEACHING NOTES:
1. Teaching Sequence — Teach this skill beginning with Phase I, then teach Phases II through IV before teaching Phase V, Steps 1 through 5, then teach Phase VI, Steps 1 through 5.
2. Phase I through IV require the student to

be able to paste paper on another sheet of paper in a random fashion whereas Phases V and VI requires the pasting of paper within prescribed boundaries.
3. Unless the student can already squeeze glue or paste from a bottle, it is suggested that some glue or paste be placed in a small container so that the student can dip the glue or paste with a stick or brush. Another alternative that is useful with physically impaired students is to use a rub-on glue stick.
4. This is a reverse chain sequence; therefore,
    a. the teacher assists the student in the performance of all phases listed after the prescribed phase. The degree of assistance is usually physical.
    b. the student completes the prescribed phase as described.
    c. the student independently completes all phases before the prescribed phase.

Fine Motor Skills

W. Uses Tongs to Pick Up Objects

Approximate Age for
Skill Acquisition
2½-3½ years

TERMINAL OBJECTIVE:	Student uses tongs to pick up a small heavy object and holds object for five seconds.
PREREQUISITE SKILLS:	Ability to grasp with thumbs and fingertips.
Phase I	Student holds tongs with hand.
Phase II	Student opens and closes tongs.
Phase III	Student picks up thick wad of cotton.
Phase IV	Student picks up large marshmallow.
Phase V	Student picks up 1-inch cube.
Phase VI	Student picks up small heavy object.

The following steps are to be used with Phases III through VI:

Steps

1. Student holds for two seconds.
2. Student holds for three seconds.

SUGGESTED MATERIALS: Tongs with action and hinges similar to scissors; 2 by 2 inch piece of cotton; large marshmallow; 1-inch cube or block; small piece of metal or other heavy object.

TEACHING NOTES:
1. Teaching Sequence — Teach this skill beginning with Phase I, then teach Phase II. Then teach Phase III, Steps 1 and 2 before teaching Phase IV, Steps 1 and 2. Continue to teach remaining phases and steps in the same manner.

X. Cuts with Scissors

Approximate Age for
Skill Acquisition
2½-3½ years

TERMINAL OBJECTIVE:	Student cuts out 20 inch circumference circle on pencil mark width border by holding paper and cutting with single-handle, blunt scissors.
PREREQUISITE SKILLS:	Ability to hold tongs and pick up objects with tongs.
Phase I	Teacher assists student to pick up double-handled scissors and hold them correctly.
Phase II	Student picks up double-handled scissors. Teacher assists student to hold them correctly.
Phase III	Student picks up double-handled scissors and inserts thumb and fingers correctly in handle.
Phase IV	Student makes three cuts (any pattern) on plain paper given complete physical assistance using double-handle scissors.
Phase V	Student makes two cuts (any pattern) on plain paper given complete physical assistance using double-handle scissors; student makes third cut independently.
Phase VI	Student makes one cut (any pattern) on plain paper given complete physical assistance using double-handle scissors; student makes second and third cuts independently.
Phase VII	Student makes three cuts on plain paper (any pattern) using double-handle scissors. Teacher assists student to hold paper.
Phase VIII	Student cuts within ½ inch wide straight line by using double-handle scissors. Teacher assists student to hold paper.
Phase IX	Student cuts within ½ inch wide straight line by holding paper and using double-handle scissors.
Phase X	Student cuts within ¼ inch wide straight line by holding paper and using double-handle scissors.
Phase XI	Student cuts on pencil mark with straight line

by holding paper and using double-handle scissors.

The following steps are to be used with Phases VIII through XI only:

Steps
1. Cuts final inch on 6 inch strip of paper.
2. Cuts final 2 inches on 8 inch strip of paper.
3. Cuts final 3 inches on 6 inch strip of paper.
4. Cuts final 4 inches on 6 inch strip of paper.
5. Cuts final 5 inches on 6 inch strip of paper.
6. Cuts 6 inches on 6 inch strip of paper.

Phase XII   Student cuts within ½ inch wide circle boundary by holding paper and using double-handle scissors.

Phase XIII   Student cuts within ¼ inch wide circle boundary by holding paper and using double-handle scissors.

Phase XIV   Student cuts on pencil-width circle boundary by holding paper and using double-handle scissors.

The following steps are to be used with Phases XII through XIV:

Steps
1. Cuts final inch on 20 inch circumference circle.
2. Cuts final 2 inches on 20 inch circumference circle.
3. Cuts final 3 inches on 20 inch circumference circle.
4. Cuts final 5 inches on 20 inch circumference circle.
5. Cuts final 7 inches on 20 inch circumference circle.
6. Cuts final 9 inches on 20 inch circumference circle.
7. Cuts final 11 inches on 20 inch circumference circle.
8. Cuts final 14 inches on 20 inch circumference circle.
9. Cuts final 17 inches on 20 inch circumference circle.
10. Cuts entire circle.

Phase XV   Student cuts 20 inch circumference circle with pencil width border by holding paper and cutting with single handle scissors.

Suggested Materials: Double-handled scissors, single-handled scissors, and stiff paper, such as construction paper. Circles are 6 inches in diameter, with varying width borders (see phases).

TEACHING NOTES:

1. Teaching Sequence — Teach this skill beginning with Phase I. Then teach Phases II through VII before teaching Phase VIII, Steps 1 through 6. Then teach Phase IX, Steps 1 through 6. Continue to teach X and XI in the same manner. Then teach Phase XII, Steps 1 through 10. Finally teach Phase XIII, Steps 1 through 10 and Phase XIV, Steps 1 through 10 before teaching Phase XV.

2. The steps in this sequence are to be taught in reverse chain. To do this, the teacher needs to assist the student to the point where he is to work independently. To aid in this process and to facilitate use of a correction procedure where the adult assists the student to perform the task, double-handled scissors are used through all but the last phase of the sequence. The last phase uses single-handled scissors and should serve to familiarize the student with the type of scissors he will be using when teaching is completed.

3. The use of double-handled scissors throughout the program is to facilitate correction of errors and does not indicate that adult is to provide complete assistance on each step.

Y. Laces Ten-Hole Card

Approximate Age for
Skill Acquisition
3-4 years

TERMINAL OBJECTIVE: Student will lace a ten-hole lacing card with a circular pattern and holes that are ⅛ inch in diameter using an alternate up and down pattern.

PREREQUISITE SKILLS: Neat pincer grasp.

Phase I — Student pulls lace tight after lace is pushed through third hole from top of card.

Phase II — Student puts tip of lace through third hold from bottom of card.

Phase III — Student pulls lace tight after lace is pushed through second hole from bottom of card.

Phase IV — Student puts tip of lace through second hole from top of card.

Phase V — Student pulls lace through first hole from top of card so that knot is against bottom of card.

Phase VI — Student puts tip of lace through first hole from bottom.

The following steps are to be used with Phases I through VI:

Steps

1. Size of hole is ½ inch; pattern of holes is a straight line. Student laces, using lacing card with three holes with ½-inch diameter placed ½ inch apart.

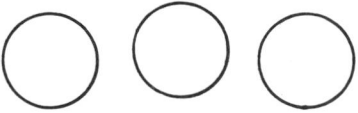

2. Size of hole is ¼ inch; pattern of holes is a straight line. Student laces, using lacing card with three holes with ¼-inch diameter placed ½ inch apart.

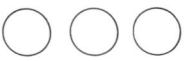

3. Size of hole is ⅛ inch; pattern is a straight line. Student laces, using

lacing card with three holes with ⅛-inch diameter placed ¼ inch apart.

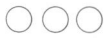

Phase VII   Student laces a ten-hole lacing card with ⅛-inch holes placed ¼ inch apart. Size of hole is ⅛ inch. Pattern is a circle.

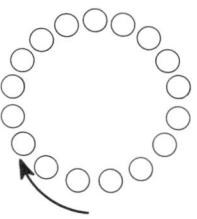

The following steps are to be used with Phase VII:

Steps
1. Student completes the tenth hole.
2. Student completes the eighth through the tenth holes.
3. Student completes the sixth through the tenth holes.
4. Student completes the fourth through the tenth holes.
5. Student completes the second through the tenth holes.
6. Student completes all ten holes.

SUGGESTED MATERIALS: Shoelace with one knotted end, cardboard or plastic foam lacing cards with patterns and hole sizes listed in the phases. For Phase VII a variety of patterns may be used.

TEACHING NOTES:
1. Teaching Sequence — Teach this skill beginning with Phase I, Step 1 before teaching Phase II, Step 1. Then teach Phases III-VI, Step 1 before teaching Phases I-VI, Step 2. Teach remaining step in the same manner.
2. This is a reverse chain sequence; therefore,
   a. the teacher assists the student in the performance of all phases listed after the prescribed phase. The degree of assistance is usually physical.
   b. the student completes the prescribed phase as described.

c. the student independently completes all phases before the prescribed phase.
3. When using the large-holed lacing cards, the adult will need to tie a large enough knot so that the end of lace is not pulled through.
4. In this sequence, lacing is done in an alternating up/down fashion, i.e. the string does *not* loop over the edge of the card.

GLOSSARY

ABDUCTION. Movement of limb outwards away from the body

ACTIVE MOVEMENTS. Movements a student does without help

ASSOCIATED REACTIONS. Increase of stiffness in spastic arms and legs resulting from effort

ASYMMETRICAL. One side of the body different from the other, unequal

ATAXIC. No balance, jerky

ATHETOID. Student with uncontrolled and continuously unwanted movements

AUTOMATIC MOVEMENTS. Necessary movements done without thought or effort

BALANCE. Not falling over, ability to keep steady position

CEREBRAL PALSY. Disorder causing diminished control of posture and movements resulting from brain damage

CLONUS. Shaky movements of spastic muscles

COORDINATION. Correct combination of muscles in movements

CONTRACTURE. Permanently tight muscles and joints

CRUISING. Side stepping, using a solid object for support

DEFORMITIES. Body or limbs fixed in abnormal positions

DIPLEGIA. Legs mostly affected

EQUILIBRIUM. Balance

EXTENSION. Straightening of trunk and limbs

FACILITATION. Making it possible for the student to move

FLEXION. Bending, as in bending of elbows, hips, knees, etc.

FLOPPY. Loose or weak posture and movements

HANDLING. Holding and moving with or without the help of the student

HALF-KNEELING. Kneeling on one knee with foot of other leg flat on floor in front of body; trunk perpendicular to floor

HEAD CONTROL. Ability to control the position of the head against gravity

HEMIPLEGIA. One side of the body affected with paralysis

INHIBITION. Positions and movements that stop muscle tightness (spasticity)

INVOLUNTARY MOVEMENTS. Unintended movements

KNEEL STAND. Kneeling with body perpendicular to floor

LATERAL. To the side

MICROCEPHALY. Very small head due to failure of the brain to grow

MIDLINE. The lengthwise center of the body

MOTIVATION. Making child want to move
MOTOR PATTERNS. The ways in which the body and limbs work together
MOVEMENT. Change of position
OCCUPATIONAL THERAPY. Treatment given to improve movements for daily living
PARAPLEGIA. Legs only affected with paralysis
PASSIVE. Without the active participation of the student, i.e. things are done *to* him without his help
PATHOLOGICAL. Abnormal
PERSEVERATION. Unnecessary repetition of movement or speech
PHYSICAL THERAPY. The treatment of disorders of movement
POSTURE. Position from which the student starts moving
PRIMITIVE MOVEMENTS. A baby's movements
PRONATION. Turning of the hand to a position with palm down
PRONE. Lying on stomach
PROTECTIVE EXTENSION. Extending arms to protect oneself from a fall in any direction
QUADRIPLEGIA. Whole body affected with paralysis
REFLEXES. Postures and movements completely out of student's control
RIGHTING. Ability to put head and body right when body positions are abnormal or uncomfortable
RIGIDITY. Very stiff movements and posture
ROTATION. Turning movement between shoulders and hips
SENSATION. Feeling
SENSORIMOTOR. Pertaining to both the senses and motor movement of the body
SIDE LYING. Lying on one's side
SIDE SITTING. Buttocks are on floor and trunk perpendicular to floor with legs bent in same direction and touching floor
SPASM. Sudden tightening of muscles
SPASTICITY. Stiffness
SUPINATION. Turning of hand to a position with palm up
SUPINE. Lying on back
SYMMETRICAL. Both sides equal
TETRAPLEGIA. All four limbs affected equally with paralysis
TONE. Firmness of muscles
TRUNK. Body
VALGUS FEET. Feet that are turned abnormally outward.
VOLUNTARY MOVEMENTS. Movements done with intention and with concentration

INDEX

A

Attains and maintains weight bearing on elbows — prone, 72
Attends to face, 52

B

Baseline, 30
Bears weight
  on elbows when placed, 66
  on extended arms — prone, 90
  on extended arms — sitting, 84
  on hands and knees when placed, 113
  on one elbow and reaches — prone, 79
  on one extended arm and reaches — hands and knees, 115
  on one knee — half-kneeling position, 167
Bracketing procedure, 26, 27
Branching, 13-15
Brings hands together — supine, 207
Builds a tower, 229

C

Crawls forward on floor, 121
Creeps
  down stairs, 176
  on hands and knees, 141
  on hands and knees, negotiating environment, 149
  up stairs, 169
Cruises, 151
Cumulative skills, 16, 25
Curricular area, 5
Curriculum, 3-20
  background and use, 3
  history of the curriculum, 3
  how the current edition was developed, 3
  how the curriculum is organized, 4
  need to maintain skills once learned, 16
  need to use support services, 16
  progression of a student through the curriculum, 12
Cuts with scissors, 242

D

Development chart, 7-11
Discrete skills, 16

F

Falls forward, 161
Fine motor skills, 203-247
Follows moving objects with eyes, 74
Forward movement — prone
  crawl forward on floor, 121
  creeps on hands and knees, 141
  creeps on hands and knees, negotiating environment, 149
  moves forward down ramp, 119
  moves toward an object, 117

G

Gets
  into a chair, 162
  up from a chair, 160
Gets to
  hands and knees, 129
  sitting from hands and knees, 130
  sitting from prone, 127
  sitting from standing, 157
  sitting from supine, 148
  standing from hands and knees, 145
Glossary, 249
Grasps
  object with both hands, 214
  two objects, one in each hand, 219
Gross motor skills, 41-202

H

Hands and knees
  bears weight on, when placed, 113
  bears weight on one extended arm and reaches, 115
  creeps on, 141
  creeps on, negotiating environment, 149
  gets to, 129
Head control
  head extension on ball, 53
  head righting on ball — prone, 70
  holds head in supported sitting, 60
  lifts head and shoulders — supine, 94
  lifts head from teacher's shoulder, 48
  lifts head — supine, 86
  lifts head while prone over bolster, 55
  maintains head control when lifted, 58

maintains head in midline — supine, 62
pulls to sit without head lag, 92
turns head — various positions, 64

I

Independent
  movement — grasp, 153
  weight bearing — grasp, 134
Intentionally releases object from grasp, 216

J

Jumps, 189

K

Kneels, 165

L

Laces ten-hole card, 245
Leans and regains balance, sitting position, 123
Lifts
  abdomen in prone position, 111
  head and shoulders — supine, 94
  head from teacher's shoulder, 48
  head — supine, 86
  head while prone over bolster, 55
  trunk with hands and arms, 139
Looks at light, 59

M

Maintains
  grasp on object — supine, 205
  head control when lifted, 58
  head in midline — supine, 205
Moves
  forward down ramp, 119
  object from one container to another, 227
  toward an object, 117

P

Pastes paper, 239
Phases, definition of, 5
Picks up
  and grasps object using neat pincer grasp, 223
  object from floor — standing, 182
Pivots on stomach, 109
Placement testing, 21-40
  general procedures, 21
  preparing for the placement test, 23
  reinforcement procedures, 30
  testing cumulative skills programs, 25
  where to begin testing, 25
Placement tests, 34-40
Posttest, 30
Probe, 31, 32
Protective extension
  falls forward, 161
  forward, 98
  forward on ball or bolster, 96
  lateral, 125
Pulls
  to kneel stand, 132
  to sitting without head lag, 92
Pushes up on extended arms — prone, 95
Puts
  cylinders in same-sized receptacle, 233
  objects in small-mouthed container, 225
  pegs in pegboard, 234
  rings on a peg, 228

R

Reaches for and picks up object
  using thumb/fingertips grasp, 221
  using whole hand grasp, 212
Reaches for
  object — prone, 211
  suspended swinging objects — supine, 209
"Red Flags" that indicate the need for support services, 19
Reverse chaining, 6, 12
Rides
  on ride-on toy, 171
  tricycle, 187
Rolling
  rolls from back to side, 88
  rolls from back to stomach, 101
  rolls from side lying to stomach, 99
  rolls from stomach to back, 81
  rolls from stomach to side, 77
  rolls side to back, 68
Running, 184

S

Sitting
  bears weight on extended arms — sitting, 84
  gets into a chair, 162
  gets to sitting from prone, 127
  gets up from a chair, 160
  holds head in supported sitting, 60
  leans and regains balance, sitting position, 123
  protective extension — lateral, 125
  seats self at table, 186
  sits in chair, 159
  sits with support, 106
  sits without support, 106
  turns trunk in sitting position, 143
Skills, definition of, 5
Stairs
  creeps down stairs, 176
  creeps up stairs, 169
  walks down stairs, 180
  walks up stairs, 178

Standing
  gets to standing from hands and knees, 145
  independent weight bearing with grasp ability, 134
  standing — no grasp ability, 137
  stands heel to toe, 198
  stands on one foot, eyes closed, 201
  stands on one foot, eyes open, 194
  stands on tiptoes, eyes closed, 199
  stands on tiptoes with eyes open, 191
  stands with support, 107
  weight bearing with ball, 103
Steps, definition of, 5
Stimulation testing, 23-25
Strings beads, 236
Support services, 16

T

Teaching notes, description of, 6
Terminal objective; definition of, 6
Tracking with eyes
  attends to face, 52
  follows moving objects with eyes, 74
  looks at light, 50
Transfers object from one hand to the other, 217
Transitions
  gets to hands and knees, 129
  gets to sitting from hands and knees, 130
  gets to sitting from prone, 127
  gets to sitting from standing, 157
  gets to sitting from supine, 148
  gets to standing from hands and knees, 145
  pulls to kneel stand, 132
  rolls from back to stomach, 101
  rolls from stomach to back, 81
Turns
  head — various positions, 64
  knob, 231
  pages of a book, one at a time, 232
  trunk in sitting position, 143

U

Unscrews and screws on jar lid, 237
Uses tongs to pick up object, 241

W

Walking
  cruising, 151
  independent movement — grasp, 153
  walking — no grasp ability, 155
  walks backward, 173
  walks down incline, 174
  walks down stairs, 180
  walks forward on a balance beam, 196
  walks up incline, 163
  walks up stairs, 178
Weight bearing
  independent — with grasp ability, 134
  with ball, 103

E3297